Depression & Natural Medicine

By Rita Elkins

Published by
Woodland Publishing Inc.
P.O. Box 160
Pleasant Grove, Utah 84062

TABLE OF CONTENTS

FORWARD

Twenty years ago a book like this would have had little chance of appearing on bookstore shelves. The notion that nutritive or herbal therapy held any value for the treatment of disease was considered a radical and irresponsible belief. Certainly, no reputable professional would have jeopardized his or her credibility by advocating the validity of non-pharmaceutical therapies.

Fortunately, today, the tide is turning. The transition may be a gradual one, but it is unquestionably in motion. The consequences of our modern society, its exposure to harmful toxins, its pitiful dietary habits and its dependence on "legitimate" drugs to survive demand that we examine the value of natural medicine.

Within the last decade, the American public has finally had the where-with-all to openly discuss its disillusionment with certain medical practices. The idea that medical science alone holds all the answers is no longer blindly accepted. Certainly, mainstream medicine saves lives. If you've been injured, need to cure a bacterial infection or require surgery for repair or replacement, traditional medicine can prove invaluable.

On the other hand, when it comes to treatment and management of allergies, degenerative diseases and mental illness, the medical establishment has a long way to go. Obviously, while no one would want to abandon the life saving technology that modern medicine affords, the medical theocracy that shuns preventative and well founded natural medicine needs to re-evaluate its posture.

It was Hippocrates who admonished: "First, do no harm." Ironically, the first thing most doctors do in treating diseases like depression is to immediately employ drastic chemical treatments that frequently do a lot of harm. The plethora of Prozac, and the prescribing of enormous quantities of sleeping pills, anti-anxiety pills, and tranquilizers testify to our inability to heal ourselves without pharmaceutical stimulation.

Regarding depression, the medical establishment may assume that new antidepressant drugs offer the best possible treatment for the majority of people suffering from depression. Certainly, no one will argue with the fact that some severe cases of depression warrant drug therapy and that it can, in fact, be life saving. On the other hand, a great many people who try antidepressant drugs, stay depressed. More importantly, many who find relief, become chemically dependent to function normally.

The information in this book confronts the deplorable lack of attention given to natural treatments that could very well cure a large number of depressed people, or at least augment standard medical therapies. All too often everything that digresses from mainstream medicine is labeled as quackery. Not so.

In addition, getting to the root of why the depression exists in the first place is rarely thoroughly investigated. One of the most common complaints people have about their doctors is that they do not take the time to address concerns, questions and possible causes. We need more questions asked, more avenues explored and more open minds.

If you or someone you know suffers from depression, find out all you can about the disease, its potential causes and treatment options. The therapies discussed in this book represent viable alternatives to orthodox medicine. Although most of these natural treatments are relatively unfamiliar to most physicians, more and more of them are being used within the medical community. Most of the references, quotes and statistical data included in our discussion originated from reputable scientists and medical doctors. The diet and nutritional breakthroughs presented in this book have their basis in scientific journals and medical records.

It must be stressed that the information in this book in no way affords the reader a mandate for self-diagnosis or self treatment. By all means, see your doctor if you feel depressed, but make sure your physician is well versed on both the conventional and alternative therapies available to you. This book will hopefully serve as a spring board from which you and your doctor can plan the best and safest treatment suitable to your particular, individual needs. Unquestionably, the 21st century medical establishment will eventually accept and practice nutritional and preventive medicine in combination with standard therapies. It's only a matter of time.

DEPRESSION:
State of Mind or State of Health?

"One cannot be deeply responsive to the world without being saddened very often."

Erich Fromm

Why are so many of us depressed? Why does a pervading sense of melancholy haunt hundreds of people, plaguing their lives with diminished purpose and performance? If you or someone you know feels depressed, you are certainly not alone. Depression is the No. 1 public health problem in the United States, and its occurrence is on the rise. One in twenty Americans develops a case of depression serious enough to require professional treatment.

While the statistics are staggering, even more shocking is the fact that depression is no longer a disorder of the middle-aged or elderly. At this writing, childhood depression is on the rise and adolescent suicide attempts are escalating. Are our lives so bleak that great numbers of our young feel compelled to waste away their lives in hopelessness or even worse, to cut them short?

The National Institute of Mental Health has estimated that over 20 million Americans may be suffering from serious depression at any given time. In addition, millions more suffer from serious mood and anxiety disorders. Why do so many of us feel like we're losing control or even worse, losing our lives?

Unquestionably, untreated depression can lead to suicide, which is the ninth leading cause of death in this country and the third leading cause in teenagers. Everyday, 15 people between the ages of 15 and 24 kill themselves. For thousands of people, doing away with themselves has become an acceptable method of escape and resolution. Anyone who has entertained the thought of suicide, even if just momentarily, needs help in confronting their depression. Keep in mind that if someone you know has made even the most casual reference to suicide, it should be taken seriously.

Perhaps, the most alarming aspect of depression is that doctors frequently fail to recognize and treat depression effectively. Moreover, while antidepressant drugs help some victims of this disease, they come with significant side-effects which are often overlooked or minimized by physicians who prescribe them.

The quickness with which conventional doctors prescribe hundreds of drugs and the magnitude of pharmaceutical usage is staggering, to say the least. Dr. Peter Briggin in *Toxic Psychiatry* states:

> *"...minor tranquilizers, barbiturates, opiates, alcohol and perhaps antidepressant's effects are short lived, with little or no evidence for sustained relief, and the hazards are considerable, including addiction, withdrawal reactions, rebound anxiety, mental dysfunction and lethality...Few psychiatrists would keep a pitcher of martinis at hand in the office to ease the anxiety of their patients; yet most are willing to reach into the drawer for a sample of `alcohol in a pill', the minor tranquilizers. Both...accomplish the same thing - a brief escape from intense feelings by suppressing or sedating normal brain function...should doctors endorse this dangerous and self-defeating avenue as a form of medical treatment?"[1]*

We live in a society which is quick to medicate itself without looking into the whys and wherefores of disease. Certainly, modern medicine saves countless lives through the use of technology and pharmaceuticals. No one's going to argue with that. It is true, however, that most alternative methods of disease treatment are thrown out all together as being nothing more than quackery, which epitomizes "throwing the baby out with the bath water."

It is unfortunate that in our vigorous attempt to treat the devastating disease of depression with the latest drugs, many of us have overlooked the profound impact of therapies which utilize diet, vitamins, amino acids, herbal preparations, light and exercise.

CONVENTIONAL MEDICINE VERSUS HOLISTIC MEDICINE

Natural medicine has traditionally been lumped in a very undesirable category by the medical profession. As a result, pertinent data and facts regarding viable treatment options frequently elude the patient. For this reason, books and articles which provide credible treatment options are invaluable to the lay person, who must learn to not only trust the medical profession, but their own ability to evaluate treatments as well.

The tried and true principles of natural healing are nothing new. For centuries they have been based on:

1. the healing power of nature,
2. doing no harm to the patient
3. identifying and treating the cause of disease not just its symptoms
4. promoting the role of physician as teacher as well as healer

The conflicting healing approaches of traditional medicine and natural medicine are striking in their opposition. As you compare the two healing philosophies, contemplate the ramifications of depressive illness. Which ideology would provide for optimal, and long lasting healing?

Standard Medical Approach		**Natural Healing**
The body is made of separate units	vs.	The body is a whole unit
Body and Mind are separate entities	vs.	Body and mind are linked
Treat the symptoms of disease	vs.	Find the cause for illness
Try to eradicate disease	vs.	Promote health
Use drugs and surgery	vs.	Address diet and lifestyle
Physicians cannot be emotionally involved	vs.	Caring is vital to healing
Physicians have the last word	vs.	Doctors work with patients
Physician controls	vs.	The patient is in charge
Focus on the objective	vs.	Focus on the subjective

Nutritional and holistic medicine incorporates the philosophy paradigm listed for natural healing. As time passes, its healing criterion is consistently being vindicated. Currently, there is a flood of new data based on continuing research in the field of nutritional medicine. To be sure, 21st century consumers will be demanding more from the medical profession in terms of natural, non-toxic treatment options for disease.

Depression is one of those disorders that can be directly linked with our overall health status as determined by our diet, among other things. If you're feeling down in the dumps, has anyone suggested that you look at what you're eating? Probably not.

It's troubling, to say the least, that present medical school criteria is sadly deficient in nutritional education. Consequently, because this particular approach to treating disease is considered a separate field, most doctors will discourage you from trying supplements or herbs. Most doesn't mean all. There is a growing contingency of medical doctors who advocate nutritional medicine. You just have to find one.

Dr. Malcolm Todd, past president of the American Medical Association put it best when he said: "Thus far physicians have shown little objective interest in promoting health and preventive care. We actually have a disease oriented cure system, rather than a health oriented care system in this country today." Looking at what we eat and how it affects our minds may be the most badly neglected area of both preventative and therapeutic medicine today.

Depression is just one of many diseases which most physicians fail to connect to dietary habits. For example, there is very little that has been published in medical literature which explores the treatment of depression with amino acids or B-vitamins. The fact remains that depression can respond favorably to these natural therapies. It only makes sense if you're feeling depressed, to inform yourself as to what's out there. Your first priority should be to find a reputable, open minded physician.

I know what you're thinking. It's true. If you feel depressed, you're not going to want to go shopping for the right doctor. Do it anyway. It's well worth the effort. Check local medical societies that may list physicians who use nutritional medicine or orthomolecular psychiatry. The Huxley Institute for Biosocial Research in Boca Raton, Florida may also be able to supply you with the names of doctors who specialize in nutritional medicine. Read on and valuable addresses will be provided which can help you track down the right doctor.

It is vital that you find a nutritionally oriented physician who will be willing to discuss the information contained in this book. Before making an appointment, ask the doctor or his receptionist if he or she is willing to use vitamins or amino acids as treatments. It may take several calls and inquiries to find a good reputable doctor who believes that nutritional therapies are sound.

When you first see your doctor, clearly explain that you would like to get over your depression without the need for potentially toxic drugs. Talk about alternative therapies that you believe would be benefit you most, and then ask him to help you implement whatever strategy you choose.

Increasing numbers of medical doctors are becoming intrigued by alternative forms of treatment. Believe it or not, there are several out there who have openly praised the advantages of natural treatments over pharmaceutical drugs. Depression is one of those diseases that can favorably respond to the types of holistic treatments discussed in this book.

The natural therapies explored in our discussion do not have the undesirable side-effects of most drugs and can offer the depressed person viable options in controlling this devastating disease. They are based on sound scientific principles and reliable data.

Contrary to popular belief, antidepressant drugs, commonly used for depression, do not provide relief for everyone who is depressed. Despite the availability of these pharmaceutical products, depression and suicide seem to be on the increase.

Keep in mind that the use of any natural therapy takes time and patience. Don't expect to see overnight results. Any good therapy takes time to implement. Using natural medicine to treat depression works best when it is combined with counseling, which can come from a doctor, a self help group, or a psychotherapist.

This book not only explores nutritional therapies but has selected various other natural methods of treating depression which are considered effective. It addresses environmental and lifestyle factors that profoundly effect how we feel and behave.

The success of natural treatments for depression depends on the individual's willingness to learn what and how to eat, to investigate unique family predispositions, and to be open to supplementation and other alternative treatments. It relies on our willingness to change our mind-set through meditation, relaxation and positive thinking.

Above all, it hinges on our ability to see ourselves as complex chemical beings subject to various ills that do indeed affect our ability to be happy. In other words, we have to develop a keen sensitivity to our biochemical selves and learn how that biochemistry affects our behavior. There are several, natural ways to change the biochemical makeup of your brain.

It would be nothing short of criminal if you believed that drug therapy was your only salvation from depression, when, in reality, your state of physical health was causing you to feel so "blah." Let's be real for a moment. Do we really know how to protect ourselves from disease by living a preventative lifestyle, or do we wait until we're sick and then pop pills without asking ourselves, "why?"

Most of us have assumed that vitamin supplements are really unnecessary and a waste of money. We routinely crave and eat chocolate and sugar to boost our ever sagging energy levels. We scoff at the idea of food allergies and treat ourselves to drinks loaded with caffeine during our breaks just to keep us going. If, somewhere along the line, we become continuously "blue", will we relate our melancholia to any of the above factors? More importantly, will our doctors address how we live as possible causes of our depressive illness?

If you are depressed and seek professional help, you are rarely asked questions like, "do you have consistent food cravings,"... do you spend a great deal of time in light deprived environments,"... or... "does your diet provide adequate sources of B vitamins." It only stands to reason that if depression is a biochemical disorder, what you put into your body does, in fact, influence its development and possible treatment.

Most health care professionals are quick to turn to anti-depressant drugs and psychotherapy in search of the quickest cure for depression. While both of these approaches can be quite effective, the role of diet, amino acids, herbs etc. should not be overlooked in the process.

Before you consider using any of these treatments, consult your doctor, who is hopefully in tune with natural health care alternatives. If you are currently on prescription medication for depression, do not discontinue or modify your dosage in any way without your doctor's supervision. Take this book with you when you see your physician and tell him you want to try natural therapies. Be assertive about your decision to try to get well naturally.

A MODERN DAY PLAGUE

"Those who do not find some time every day for health must sacrifice a lot of time one day for illness."

Sebastian Kneipp

Depression, like so many modern day diseases has reached epidemic proportions since World War II. Why? While the disease has been with us since the beginning of recorded history, the unprecedented number of depressed people within this generation is alarming. What's happening to us and our children? It has only been within the last few years that depression has been linked to a biochemical imbalance in the brain. In the past, depressed individuals were terribly misunderstood, stigmatized, and treated with a host of bizarre therapies, including bloodletting and exorcism. Clearly, today treatments have improved, however, the question as to why depression is so prevalent remains.

The sheer numbers of depressed people earns depression the title of a modern day plague. Estimates indicate that up to 15% of the U.S. population will become a victim of depression before they hit the age of 40. More than twice as many women are presently undergoing some form of therapy for depression than men. The enormous consumption of Prozac, one of the most widely prescribed drugs for depression, has hit the front page and continues to spawn controversy. Regardless of its supposed link with abnormal behavior, Prozac continues to remain the nation's best-selling antidepressant.

While it is generally accepted that women are more prone to becoming depressed, men tend to deny that they get depressed but, of course, they do. Geriatric depression exists in epidemic proportions. People over 65 are much more likely to become depressed than the rest of the population. Depression among older segments of our population has skyrocketed over the last few years.

Advocates for the elderly are literally begging doctors to re-evaluate the horrific over-medication of senior citizens. Many strongly believe

that the overwhelming amount of drugs prescribed to our elderly is what's making them act "goofy," not senility or depression.

Most professionals attribute the dreadful numbers of people who have become depressed to various maladies of twentieth-century living. While they view the disease as a liability of modern, fast-paced life, they frequently ignore the very catalysts to depression that can be managed or controlled.

The question is: are we overlooking possible causal factors in our ardor to find a quick cure for this malady. Has the role of hormones, carbohydrates, excessive dieting, light deprivation or the psychogenic effects of hundreds of widely prescribed drugs been sufficiently investigated? In our zeal to cure ourselves, have we been overlooking the very things that may greatly enhance our ability to eliminate or even avoid depression?

BABY BOOMERS AND DEPRESSION

Several studies show that the incidence of depression has been dramatically increasing among people who were born after 1940. Baby boomers are much more likely to become depressed than people who were born before 1940. What's going on? Some experts have theorized that the reason we have more depression is because more people are aware of the disease, therefore it is more often reported than in previous years. It is more likely, however, that post World War II lifestyles have increasingly demanded more from successive generations and offered less in terms of good nutrition and emotional support.

It is also true that pollution, poor eating habits, eating disorders and spending time in closed, badly lit and ventilated environments have also escalated since the 1940's. Eating disorders afflict enormous numbers of young women. In addition, eating overly processed fast foods and highly sugared foods has become the rule rather than the exception. Much of the food we consume today has been fragmented, chemically altered and unnaturally preserved. In addition, we're now eating non-food substitutes as if they were the real thing. Aspartane, saccharine, fake fats, artificial textures, colors etc. are casually ingested with no real thought given to their long term effects. Most of us assume if the FDA says it's OK, then it is.

As mentioned earlier, adolescent depression has dramatically escalated over the last few decades. Suicide is the third leading cause of

death for teenagers. Among college students, it's the second leading cause of death. It is estimated that over 5000 teenagers commit suicide every year. Between the years of 1970 and 1978, the suicide rate for those between the ages of 15 and 24 rose forty-one percent.[2]

One of the most shocking facts to come out of studies of teenage suicides was that most of these teens had deplorable eating habits and in many ways were malnourished. A typical teenager exists on caffeine, white sugar, alcohol, drugs and high fat, empty calorie junk foods. Sound scientific facts back up the fact that without certain nutrients, the brain cannot function normally. It's not difficult to see that this type of diet would have disastrous implications for the human body and mind.

Moreover, adolescence is an extremely stressful time. Stress can leach out nutrients from the body with the B-vitamins being particularly vulnerable. Eating disorders and starvation diets are common behaviors among our young women. Being thin is a terrible stressor and promotes extreme dieting, which results in nutrient depletions causing more emotional stress. This vicious cycle of stress and vitamin depletion can continually wear down resistance and produce mood alteration. It's a malicious predicament. The lower our levels of nutrients become, the less able we are to cope with stress....the more stress we experience, the lower our level of nutrients become.

The implications of the typical American diet on emotional and mental health are staggering to say the least. If seventy-five percent of the deaths in this country are due to lifestyle-related diseases, what percent of mental illness is directly influenced by the same factors as well? No one really knows at this point. We're just beginning to see the tip of the iceberg when it comes to lifestyle and its relationship to mood disorders.

There is no question that a lack of the proper nutrients can profoundly affect mood and mental outlook. Inadequate nutrition among our youth may be exacting an ominous toll in the form of depression and suicide. Certainly, factors such as peer pressure, grades, money problems and family stressors have to be considered. It must be realized, however, that without adequate nutrition, these challenges are compounded. In other words, if you become deficient in certain nutrients, your ability to cope is greatly impaired. In fact, your vision of reality may be significantly distorted.

The break-up of the traditional family unit has also been cited as a possible component in fostering depression. Family stability for many of us is a thing of the past. Spiritual issues have largely been neglected and put on the back burner within the last thirty years. The result can be a futile search for a very elusive kind of happiness.

Our nation has experienced a spiritual famine. Discussing or utilizing religion in public forums has become prohibited. Certainly, a lack of spiritual focus only contributes to feelings of dissatisfaction and frustration. For generations, holistic medicine has taught that man cannot be truly healthy or happy for that matter, unless all parts of his being are nourished. In many ways, the emotional and spiritual facets of our society have been badly abused and even worse, ignored.

Remember, however, that it's almost impossible to feel happy, regardless of your circumstances or spiritual orientation, if you are not getting enough of certain key nutrients. It has to be acknowledged that our physical state, determined by what we eat, the drugs we take, and what we are exposed to in terms of pollution, light, stress etc. plays a profound role in controlling our moods and mental outlook.

Unfortunately, many of us minimize the dramatic impact that diet, natural medicine and alternative treatments can offer victims of depression. We are frequently prone to believing that drug therapy is the only effective method of treating this disorder. In so doing, we often overlook lifestyle practices and alternative treatments that could literally work wonders for people who suffer from mood disorders.

For example, changing what you eat and when you eat it may have a pivotal impact on mood swings. The role of sugar, caffeine, cholesterol, vitamins, amino acids, herbs, and light, should not be underestimated in their impact. These factors can adversely affect mood and influence behavior. Most of us who have struggled to control melancholia rarely consider these hidden, everyday catalysts to depression.

Moreover, it must be understood that depression can be a by-product of a number of abnormal conditions. Yeast infections, viruses, a faulty thyroid gland and exposure to toxic chemicals can create depression in certain individuals and should be addressed as possible causal factors in both its treatment and prevention.

Ironically, nineteenth-century doctors viewed depression as the result of chemical imbalances, an idea that was thrown out by Freud and Jung who categorized depression as a psychological disease created by an over-active conscience. The present scientific trend supports the notion that biochemistry and genetic predisposition can cause depression in combination with certain psychological factors. In other words, certain experiences for certain people can trigger the type of change in brain chemistry that can make you feel sad.

As a result, most professionals will treat depression both physically and psychologically. The availability of several anti depressant drugs reiterates the very real connection between chemistry and mood. Undoubtedly, these drugs can help certain individuals, however, their side-effects should be thoroughly discussed. The premise of this book is that valuable treatment tools also exist in areas of nutrition and health promoting therapies which are much safer and, in some cases, more effective than drugs. Becoming aware of what's out there and how it works is the key.

THE DELICATE BIOCHEMICAL EQUILIBRUIUM OF MOOD

The most dramatic discovery in putting together the research for this book was learning that the interrelationship between sugar, hormones, light, exercise, B-vitamins and certain amino acids was intrinsically involved in a complex chemical feedback loop, which seems to intensify in many people who suffer from depression.

In other words, the puzzle is beginning to come together. Research is proving that in a large number of cases, physical reasons exist which determine emotional response, reasons that are interwoven in complex biochemical reactions. The delicate nature of these chemical balances in the brain seems particularly susceptible to dietary habits.

Be assured that as soon as proper chemical balances are achieved in the brain, your attitude toward life will change. Coping skills will improve, optimism will return and physical as well as psychological health will dramatically improve.

From 1960 to 1989, the cost of health care in America escalated from $27 billion to $500 billion dollars and is still rising. Much of the money spent for health care went to treating diseases which are the by-product of bad eating habits and lack of exercise. While medical science has recognized heart disease and cancer as life-style related disorders, mental disorders have been viewed from a different angle. It's time to change that perception.

Hopefully, the information contained in this book may shed new light on depression, a disease which is currently a national health crisis and threatens to make most of us dependent on drugs to feel good. The goal of this book is to inform those who suffer from depression, that there are natural treatments available, which should ideally be tried with the cooperation of your physician. We, as individuals must take responsibility for gathering information that will enable us to make educated choices about our own health care.

It's up to you to investigate the facts and draw your own conclusions. Knowledge is empowerment. The premise of this book is that in many instances, you can control your moods through natural therapies and live a rich, safe, healthy and happy life.

ARE YOU DEPRESSED?

"I've developed a new philosophy...I only dread one day at a time."

Charlie Brown

I strongly believe that at certain times in my life I have been seriously depressed and didn't even know it. Sometimes, I would go for weeks on end hiding in my house, alternating between gloomy and not so gloomy, assuming that certain flaws in my personality were responsible. How many of us were raised in households where the mood of one or both of our parents determined whether it would be a good day or a bad one? Did our parents know how to recognize depression? Are we in a position to identify depressive illness for what it really is? Frequently, we mistake depression for chronic fatigue or other disorders which are discussed further in a later section of this book. Being depressed sounds pretty ominous, and many of us think that we have to feel suicidal in order to be considered clinically "depressed."

On the contrary, if you experience sudden mood changes that create dramatic swings in your feelings or struggle with persistent or periodic changes in mood, you may be suffering from depression. If you're down in the dumps more than you're up enjoying life, you are probably suffering from some form of depressive illness. Everyone feels blue at one time or another. This is a fact of life here on earth. The normalcy of occasional low moods makes it difficult to distinguish a true melancholia from just a normal emotional slump. When sad feelings last and intensify, or periodically appear for no good reason, or if you've forgotten how to be happy, its time to take some action.

Occasionally, we all get the "blahs." It must be understood, however, that feeling blue from time to time and being depressed are not the same thing. True depression is a disorder and not a normal part of everyday living. It strikes people of all nationalities, backgrounds and ages. Understandably, various life events can precipitate a period of depression. In a vast number of cases, however, depression develops for no apparent reason.

Technically, there are two types of depression: reactive and endogenous. Reactive depression typically results from a particular situation such as the death of a loved one, marital discord or financial difficulties. People who have this form of depression will usually improve with time and may benefit from psychotherapy as well.

On the other hand, people with endogenous depression, which cannot be linked to any specific event, frequently fail to respond to psychotherapy and find themselves unable to break out of their mental misery. If you fall into this category of depression, brain biochemistry may be the culprit. If this is the case, it's up to you to take the necessary steps to help yourself.

People who suffer from a mild biochemical imbalance may only experience sporadic symptoms of mild depression. If, however, they are thrown into a serious emotional crisis, they may become prone to severe depression. In these instances, depression is the result of a combination of reactive and endogenous factors. Before you can take any therapeutic approach, you need to determine if you are truly depressed.

HOW YOU FEEL WHEN YOU'RE DEPRESSED

When you feel depressed you usually hate yourself and everyone else. It's difficult to concentrate when your feel low, and even simple decisions can seem overwhelming. Feelings of frustration, hopelessness, and lethargy are common to depression. If you are a woman, you have the added challenge of hormonal factors, which can further aggravate and intensify mood swings.

Elayne Boosler says that when women get depressed they either eat or go shopping. Men, on the other hand, invade other countries. It's a whole different way of thinking. While there may be both humor and truth in her assessment, women who are seriously depressed usually don't even feel like spending money. Depression can make you react a number of ways, all of which are negative.

A depresssed mind-set produces thoughts like these: " I'm so tired all the time...I just can't take any of this....nothing is left that makes life worth living...every task, even something as simple as getting dressed has become incredibly hard...I need to run away and escape, but there's no where to go, or even worse, there is no one that understands how I feel...nothing matters, nothing."

Typically, depression makes you feel dismal for several weeks on end. It makes pleasurable experiences like eating or being romantic seem empty and unsatisfying. Depression can make you feel like you're in slow motion and even small tasks become monumental ones. Depression fills its victims with self-doubt and makes them feel perpetually pessimistic about their futures. Depression drains energy and fills the mind with thoughts of self-destruction.

The characteristic attitude of a depressed individual spawns thoughts and feelings that are never conducive to self-improvement or productivity. Such thoughts may include:

- Life is a hopeless trip to nowhere.
- The world is a horrible place to have to live.
- I have no friends and I don't really want any I don't like people.
- Why doesn't anything seem fun or interesting anymore?
- I wish I could just sleep time away.
- I'm always tired and mornings are the worst time of the day.
- Even when I'm with people, I feel terribly lonely.
- I wish I could escape myself.

If you have experienced any of these feelings, you have probably been depressed and may have even contemplated suicide. Be assured that there is plenty to live for and that states of depression can be cured and do pass. What's even more encouraging, if you experience periodic mood swings, you may be able to effectively control "down" times through dietary management alone. The important thing is that you see your doctor right away and begin to unravel your depression.

If you or anyone you know is experiencing any of the following signs, see a doctor as soon as possible or call a suicide help number.

WARNING SIGNS OF SUICIDE

- FAMILY HISTORY OF SUICIDE OR ANY PREVIOUS SUICIDE ATTEMPT
- OVERWHELMING FEELINGS OF HOPELESSNESS
- WITHDRAWAL FROM EVERYDAY ACTIVITIES
- SOCIAL ISOLATION THAT IS USUALLY SELF-IMPOSED
- DRASTIC MOOD SWINGS OR PERSONALITY CHANGES
- NEGLECTING PERSONAL HYGIENE, FINANCES, PETS ETC.
- WEIGHT CHANGES
- RECENT TRAUMA
- GIVING AWAY PERSONAL POSSESSIONS, PUTTING AFFAIRS IN ORDER
- SUDDEN CALM OR UPLIFTED MOOD AFTER PERIOD OF DEPRESSION
- BUYING A GUN
- VERBAL OR WRITTEN REFERENCES TO SUICIDE
- FREQUENT DRUG OR ALCOHOL USE

Depression that is continuous and overwhelming in its impact is a life-threatening disease that slowly destroys its victims and sometimes renders family and friends helpless. It invades every facet of one's life and regardless of spiritual affiliation, can sometimes succeed in totally incapacitating or destroying its victims.

It is easy to mistake depression for other ailments. If, for example you are experiencing chronic, unexplained aches and pains or consistent digestive disturbances, you might be, in fact, depressed. Frequently, depression can masquerade as persistent headaches, backaches, muscle spasms, sleep disturbances, chronic fatigue, constipation or changes in weight.

Being constantly worried, overly anxious or concerned about everyday things can also mean that you're depressed. If you find yourself repeatedly waking up in the middle of the night and working yourself up into a frenzy over what are really very manageable stressors, you may be reacting to a disruption in brain biochemistry that causes depression.

It's typical, when you're depressed to be plagued with persistent negative thoughts and phobias, which predispose you to all kinds of exaggerated fears and anxieties. You many spend a whole night stewing about something as simple as getting your car registration in on time to worrying about the potential threat of an earthquake.

Along with other symptoms, when you're depressed, you feel on edge, high strung or prone to panicky feelings for no apparent reason. Often depression makes us feel unusually phobic about seemingly harmless situations. You may have driven across town to do some shopping and suddenly feel terror stricken because you're so far from home. If something like this happens, you may decide to see your doctor, who will probably begin drug therapy for panic disorders, possibly missing all together that your panic disorder stems from a depressive illness.

Although less common, doing wild, implusive things like spending a great deal of money on trivial items or drastically altering your appearance can also be signs of a mood disorder. Frequently, because decision making becomes so difficult when you feel depressed, bad decisions may occur, compounding feelings of low self-esteem. Something like picking the wrong entree off of a menu may seem like a devastating disappointment.

Sometimes, if you've battled depression for an extended period of time, a small irritation can be seen as an enormous calamity. A family friend, who fell prey to this faulty perception of reality, committed suicide one Sunday morning after the towel rack in his bathroom fell off the wall. In his mind, this seemingly insignificant event, toppled a whole mountain of emotional stressors and literally pushed him over the edge.

The majority of depressed people suffer from the inability to enjoy anything and experience a pervasive feeling of fatigue. If you have at least four of the following symptoms which have persisted for two weeks or more, you may be suffering from clinical depression:

- A FEELING OF PERSISTENT SORROW, EMPTINESS OR ANXIETY
- EXCESSIVE CRYING
- EXPERIENCING PHOBIC BEHAVIOR SUCH A FEAR OF BEING ALONE, OR ANXIETY ATTACKS
- FEELINGS OF HOPELESSNESS AND OVERWHELMING

PESSIMISM
- FEELINGS OF WORTHLESSNESS, HELPLESSNESS OR GUILT
- LOSS OF INTEREST OR PLEASURE IN ORDINARY ACTIVITIES, INCLUDING SEX
- SLEEP DISTURBANCES WHICH INCLUDE INSOMNIA, OVERSLEEPING OR WAKING UP TOO EARLY
- EATING DISTURBANCES WHICH INCLUDES A LOSS OR INCREASE IN APPETITE
- FATIGUE AND MALAISE OR A LOSS OF AMBITION
- RESTLESSNESS OR IRRITABILITY
- DIFFICULTY MAKING SIMPLE DECISIONS OR IN CONCENTRATING OR REMEMBERING FACTS
- HALLUCINATIONS OR DELUSIONS
- THOUGHTS OF SUICIDE, OR DEATH OR ANY ATTEMPTS AT SUICIDE

In addition, symptoms of depression in the workplace may be recognized as a decrease in productivity, an unwillingness to cooperate, a rise in safety problems, an increase in accidents, a variety of unexplained aches and pains, alcohol or drug abuse, missing school or work on a regular basis, or a persistent lack of energy. Unfortunately, there is no single, reliable test that can conclusively prove that you are suffering from depression.

The following test, known as the *Wakefield Questionnaire* used in places like the University of Wisconsin Medical School can help you assess your particular mental state and may point out some symptoms of depression that you may have overlooked.

Read each statements and then circle the number of front of the statement that best describes how you feel now, not in the past or how you hope to feel in the future.

A. I feel miserable and sad.
   (0) No, not at all
   (1) No, not much
   (2) Yes, sometimes
   (3) Yes, definitely

B. I find it easy to do the things I used to do.
(0) Yes, definitely
(1) Yes, sometimes
(2) No, not much
(3) No, not at all

C. I get a very frightened or panicky feeling for apparently no reason at all.
(0) No, not at all
(1) No, not much
(2) Yes, sometimes
(3) Yes, definitely

D. I have weeping spells, or feel like it.
(0) No, not at all
(1) No, not much
(2) Yes, sometimes
(3) Yes definitely

E. I still enjoy the things I used to.
(0) Yes, definitely
(1) No, not much
(2) Yes, sometimes
(3) Yes, definitely

F. I am restless and can't keep still.
(0) No, not at all
(1) No, not much
(2) Yes, sometimes
(3) Yes, definitely

G. I get off to sleep easily without sleeping tablets.
(0) Yes, definitely
(1) Yes, sometimes
(2) No, not much
(3) No, not at all

H. I feel anxious when I go out of the house on my own.
(0) No, not at all
(1) No, not much
(2) Yes, sometimes
(3) Yes, definitely

I. I have lost interest in things.
(0) No, not at all
(1) No, not much
(2) Yes, sometimes
(3) Yes, definitely

J. I get tired for no reason
(0) No, not at all
(1) No, not much
(2) Yes, sometimes
(3) Yes, definitely

K. I am more irritable than usual.
(0) No, not at all
(1) No, not much
(2) Yes, sometimes
(3) Yes, definitely

L. I wake early and then sleep badly for the rest of the night.
(0) No, not at all
(1) No, not much
(2) Yes, sometimes
(3) Yes, definitely

Add up the circled numbers for all twelve questions. If your score is 15 or higher, you should make an appointment with your doctor and show him the test. If your score was below 15, but you still feel that you might be depressed, see your doctor anyway and discuss your symptoms.

Recognizing and treating depression early can decrease the severity and length of depression. Make sure you tell your physician that you would like to explore natural treatments before you go on antidepressant drugs. How to find a doctor who is willing to explore natural avenues of treatment is discussed in a later section of this chapter.

THE HIDDEN FACES OF DEPRESSION

While it seems far-fetched, most depressed people do not recognize the fact that they are, in fact, depressed. Consequently, they may go from doctor to doctor describing an endless list of physical symptoms which have no apparent cause. This exercise in futility can make matters worse. The more doctors you see, the more medication you'll probably take, while the source of the problem remains undiscovered.

In some cases, like the panic disorder we cited earlier, specific symptoms may be treated and even relieved, however the underlying cause can often escape both patient and doctor. For example, Chronic Fatigue Syndrome may be, in reality, depression disguised as a consistent feeling of exhaustion. Likewise, a serious loss in appetite, insomnia or a decrease in weight may not be attributed even by the most qualified diagnostician as side-effects of the primary problem: depression.

It is now widely accepted that depression accounts for a vast number of visits to the doctor's office, and is unfortunately, frequently misdiagnosed and treated. It turns out that in some cases, you may have a legitimate physical problem that is accompanied by a separate depression. The important thing is to distinguish the difference.

Frederick K. Goodwin, director of the National Institute for Mental Health says that doctors who don't specialize in psychiatry recognize depression in only 25 percent of cases. Even he admits that they are likely to prescribe anti-anxiety drugs or sleeping pills which can act as depressants themselves, only making matters worse.[3]

Donald F. Klein, director of research at the New York State Psychiatric Institute and co-author of the book *Understanding Depression* warns that even some psychiatrists are not up to date in treating depression..."being too wedded to lengthy psychoanalysis, perhaps, or unskilled in fine-tuning medication."[4] It's hard to believe that despite scientific evidence, the idea that depression is purely a psychological disorder still prevails in the minds of many people. Recent research suggests that this is rarely the case. If you feel consistently low or blue and you really don't have a good enough reason to feel this way, chances are, brain biochemistry is involved.

The human body operates best when all of its systems are balanced and working together in harmony. Everything that happens to us can disrupt that delicate equilibrium. As a result, we may feel unexplainably sad for prolonged periods of time. Anyone who has had surgery or suffered a significant illness may understand this concept all too well.

If you have recently had an operation or have struggled with a chronic or acute disease and you become depressed, the assumption is that you are just reacting emotionally to physical stress. What is rarely explored are the very real biochemical effects of surgery, illness or drug therapy on the brain. You may very well be depressed because of a physical phenomenon. A kind of post-traumatic stress syndrome can occur after these types of events. How many of us are aware of that fact? For a more in-depth discussion on unrecognized causes of depression, see a later chapter.

Unexplained pain can also be a marker of depression. For some people, coping with emotional crisis means channeling mental anxiety into physical ailments, a process referred to as somatizing. When this occurs, being depressed can mean that you are also experiencing a number of mysterious aches and pains. Depression makes you turn inward. In so doing, you sometimes become acutely aware of your body systems. This unnatural preoccupation with your physical state can exaggerate physical symptoms, making them appear much worse than they really are.

If you are ashamed of the possibility that you are depressed and believe that a social stigma accompanies the illness, think again. Depression is not your fault. It's a disorder like any other disorder and is never a sign of weakness or lack of discipline. Don't beat yourself up more by assuming that only losers get depressed. Depression can snag the heartiest and the best.

Don't waste time denying your depression. If you have found yourself going from doctor to doctor with puzzling physical symptoms, or if you find that you never seem to improve, consider the fact that you might be suffering from some form of depression. Get help right away. Life is too precious. There is so much to experience and to learn and so little time. Don't cheat yourself.

While this book advocates the value of natural therapies to treat depression, it is vital to find a good doctor who can assist you in deciding on treatment options. Keep in mind that even the best doctors often become preoccupied with managing symptoms rather than actually healing disease, and depression is a disease, like any other.

The first step to curing depression is to accurately diagnose the condition. Make sure your doctor is willing to try to discover the reason you feel depressed and not just put you on medication right off the bat. Good doctors will gather all the pertinent data they can in order to determine what's going on. You should be asked questions about your personal life, your dietary habits, drugs you may be taking, and your family history. Certain lab tests should be ordered to make sure that other illnesses are not involved.

FIND THE RIGHT KIND OF DOCTOR FOR YOU

Finding the right doctor is crucial. When you go for your first visit, watch for the following:

* Does your doctor listen closely and give you ample opportunity to express yourself?
* Does your doctor ask question concerning your medical history, eating habits, drug interactions, etc. etc.?
* Does your doctor seem genuinely interested in what you have to say and in treating you according to some of your own desires?
* Does your doctor respond well to your questions, no matter how trivial they may seem?
* Do you feel rushed, uncomfortable or tense in the presence of your doctor?
* Do you like and respect your doctor?

In assessing the value of seeing certain physicians, in combination with the above questions, your intuition will be of great value. Do not continue treatment with any doctor you are unsure of. Find a good one that will fulfill your needs.

If you are still seeing your family physician, ask your GP if depression may be a possibility. If he or she is unreceptive or curt, change doctors. Patricia Slagle, M.D., who suffered from depression for years, stresses that disorders like insomnia and anxiety may be the result of depression. Unfortunately, the typical scenario involves the prescription of a tranquilizing drug such as Valium, or using sleeping pills to promote what is never really "restful" sleep.

Slagle points out that "82 percent of patients who killed themselves had seen their physician within one month of their death and 55 percent died of an overdose of tranquilizing and sleep medication supplied by the doctor. It's my belief that doctors would be wise to clearly consider depression in all those with sleeping problems or anxiety and to treat them more appropriately for their depression."[5] A current report on depression from Johns Hopkins University stated that antidepressants are the fourth leading cause of drug overdose and the third leading cause of drug-related death.[6]

Most physicians will assume that your depression is either psychological, biochemical or a combination of the two. Whatever probable cause your doctor believes is making you feel depressed, any nutritionally oriented factors are usually ignored. You probably won't be asked if you have any particular food cravings or if you use caffeine or take vitamin supplements. For this reason, it is imperative that you seek out an open-minded physician who is willing to help you plan a treatment strategy based on your particular psychological and physical needs.

If you believe you are depressed, take action. You may feel helpless and hopeless, but you don't have to. Today, more than ever, depression can be successfully treated and frequently cured all together. Time is passing and there's too much living to do. Find an open minded doctor and put natural medicine to work for you.

The American Holistic Medical Association is comprised of medical doctors and osteopaths who believe in treating more than just the symptoms of disease. Write to the address below for names of physicians in your area that are members of this organization.

American Holistic Medical Association
4101 Lake Boone Trail, Suite 201
Raleigh, North Carolina 27607
919-787-5146

The American Association of Naturopathic PHysicians (AANP) is another professional organization that lists licensed naturopathic physicians in your area.

The American Association of Naturopathic Physicians
P.O. Box 20386
Seattle, WA 98102
206-323-7610

BRAIN CHEMISTRY...
_____ PREDICTOR OF MOOD

"It is often the scientist's experience that he senses the nearness of truth when connections are envisioned. A connection is a step toward simplification, unification."
Mahlon Hoagland

During the 1940's it was finally accepted that biochemical events in the body can profoundly effect behavior and mood. Subsequently, the issue of the body-brain connection was revitalized and a host of new antipsychotic, and antidepressant drugs hit the market. Even more dramatic was the discovery that correlations exist between neurotransmitters and emotional and mental behavior.

The brain requires certain chemicals to function normally. When the level of these chemicals is disrupted, depression can occur. It can be that simple. This neurochemical connection is called the monoamine theory of depression and has motivated the creation of several kinds of antidepressant drugs, which are currently prescribed to thousands of depressed individuals.

While the quantity of these brain chemicals is crucial, the sensitivity of certain receptor cells to the presence of these chemicals is also critical. After brain chemicals or neurotransmitters are released, they attach to receptor cells which are designed to link with that particular chemical alone. Imagine the chemical as a key and the receptor cell, the lock. In order for the door to be opened, the two must fit. When a fit occurs, a certain effect is produced.

For example, some neurotransmitters transmit impulses that excite, while others inhibit and minimize. Similarly, some produce positive feelings of well being, while others cause the development of negative or depressed sensations. It is important to remember that while the quantity of these chemicals is important, if the receptor cells are impaired in any way, the key is there but the lock is missing.

Endorphin is one of the more well known neurotransmitters. It has the ability to relieve pain and also produce feelings of euphoria. You're probably aware of recent research which has suggested that certain forms of sustained exercise can actually produce endorphins, which can create a new feeling of energy or well being. This reaction is typically seen in sports such as long distance running. As mentioned earlier, endorphin binds to a specific receptor cell in the brain.

Several other neurotransmitters are also responsible for regulating all brain activity and functions, which include not only mood control but memory, appetite, sleep etc. In most people suffering from depression, levels of neurotransmitters located in the mood controlling areas of the brain are abnormally low. Consequently, these signals or impulses are not transmitted fast enough to adequately sustain normal mood. Anti depressant drugs address this problem by increasing the amount of these specific brain chemicals, especially one called serotonin.

What must be asked at this point is, are there other ways to stimulate the brain's production and reservoir of these chemicals? Research strongly suggests that through natural methods, it is possible to achieve the same or similar results as those created by prescription drugs. The key lies in understanding how our bodies respond to mood changes and knowing what nutritive measures and supplements to take at the appropriate time.

In her book, *The Way Up From Down,* Priscilla Slagle, a medical doctor who suffered from chronic depression for years relates how she takes an amino acid and a vitamin if she wakes up feeling down. She writes: "It rarely happens any more these days, but if I ever awaken in the morning feeling slightly low, I take several tyrosine capsules and put a few sublingual vitamin B-12's under my tongue. Within an hour my mood and outlook will have completely improved. I don't have to waste unnecessary time and energy on an unwanted, unneeded state of being, and I experience no side-effects whatsoever."[7]

It's hard to believe that minute amounts of brain chemicals can determine the regulation of our behavior and determine our state of mind. Three of these neurotransmitters are particularly crucial in determining the way we feel about life. Certain levels of dopamine, serotonin and norepinephrine play a vital role in creating energy, optimism, and in easing tension.

At the same time, deficits in these chemicals, particularly serotonin, can generate feelings of fatigue, despair and heightened nervousness. On the other hand, too much norepinephrine can create mania, which is technically the opposite of depression.

Before we get into the specifics of natural treatments designed to restore normal brain chemistry, lets look at standard medical treatments for depressive illness.

MEDICAL VS. NATURAL OPTIONS

"I will follow that system of regimen which, according to my ability and judgement, I consider for the benefit of my patients, and abstain from whatever is deleterious..."

from the Hippocratic Oath

Not too many years ago, doctors would try to wait out depression or use stimulants such as amphetamines to artificially stimulate the nervous system. Electroconvulsive therapy, commonly called shock treatments was used in severe cases and earned a very bad reputation. ECT therapy has come a long way and some doctors believe it can now be used safely and more effectively than drugs. It's still a drastic form of therapy. Electrodes are attached to the scalp and a mild current is passed through them which can in some cases trigger unconsciousness or seizures. This therapy is usually employed in place of drugs. Using muscle relaxants and anesthetics has reduced many of the past problems associated with ECT.

In the 1950's a class of drugs known as monoamine oxidase inhibitors emerged and they were regarded as a breakthrough for depression sufferers. Unfortunately, like so many other prescription drugs, they had a whole host of undesirable side-effects.

Today, depression treatment has entered the age of the tricyclic antidepressants, which are considered significantly less risky than MOAI's (monoamine oxidase inhibitors). As mentioned earlier, antidepressant drugs work by increasing levels of serotonin and norepinephrine. As a result, mood and attitude improve. Both of these brain chemicals belong to the amine family. Remember the word amine.

The brain is designed to conserve these very vital chemicals through a process called re-uptake. This process re-uses most of the amine that has been released in the brain. The remaining amount is chemically changed by an enzyme referred to as MAO (monoamine oxidase) and is normally excreted in the urine.

While this system seems amazingly efficient in ensuring that the brain is adequately supplied with these neurotransmitters, there are several factors which can impair this mechanism. Some of these include:

- an original lack of amines which can be caused by an insufficient supply of amino acids, vitamins and minerals;
- an increased and abnormal need for the necessary chemicals needed to manufacture these amines, a condition which can be genetic;
- the receptor cells may be impaired, consequently, the amine is not received and utilized;
- the re-usage and recycling process of the brain may be impaired;
- an excess of MAO may inadvertently destroy too much of the brain's amine supply.

Interestingly, this last possibility can also be an inherited tendency.

HOW ANTIDEPRESSANT DRUGS WORK

Antidepressant drugs are designed to artificially keep an adequate supply of these amines available to brain cells. They can achieve this by blocking the re-uptake process so an increased supply of the amine will accumulate. This is how Prozac and Zoloft work. Another option is for the drug to block the action of MOA, or to increase the sensitivity of receptor cells. The class of drugs called tricyclic antidepressants (imipramine, amitriptyline, desipramine, etc.) works by preventing serotonin and norepinephrine from returning to the nerve cell that released them. In this way their effect is amplified.

Drug therapy for depression can be quite effective, however, antidepressants can provoke a host of side-effects. Most doctors will hop on the drug bandwagon and may even neglect to discuss side-effects, which are usually referred to as minor. It is also important to realize that although drugs provide relief in many cases, as many as 30 percent of depressed people fail to respond favorably to even the newest pharmaceuticals available.

If you are depressed, you are usually told you only have one choice: to weigh the risk of drug side-effects against the risk of the disease itself. Tricyclic antidepressants can produce adverse reactions in the cardiovascular system, including rapid heartbeat, high blood pressure, palpitations, abnormal heart rhythms and in some cases, heart attack and stroke. Psychiatric reactions include: hallucinations, confusion, anxiety, nightmares, insomnia and disorientation.

In addition, the tricyclic family of antidepressants can also cause numbness, tingling, loss of coordination, ringing in the ears and seizures. If the drug is abruptly discontinued, nausea, headache and malaise may occur.

Antidepressant drugs should be administered with extreme caution to anyone who suffers from epilepsy, Parkinson's disease, heart problems, glaucoma, high blood pressure, liver disorders and to anyone with urinary disorders. Overdosing on an antidepressant drug can be fatal. Priscilla Slagle, M.D. points out that a number of depressed people will commit suicide with their antidepressant drug.[8]

The monoamine oxidase inhibitor class of drugs has similar

side-effects as the tricyclics. One of the more serious side effects from these antidepressants is called hypertensive crisis, which occurs when the blood pressure climbs so high that it may trigger bleeding in the brain. The threat of serious hypertension also exists if a person taking this type of drug eats foods which contain an amine called tyramine which includes: aged cheese, wine, yogurt, yeast extract, liver, some beans, chocolate and caffeine.

Of particular interest is the fact that one of the MOA inhibitor antidepressant drugs called phenelzine sulfate (Nardil) can inhibit the action of vitamin B-6 which is especially effective in maintaining good mental health. Ironically, prolonged use of this drug may cause a lack of this vitamin, which in itself can cause depression.

Newer antidepressant medications such as trazodone and maprotiline hydrochloride have less side-effects than the MOA inhibitors, however, they are certainly not without their potential drawbacks. While the benefits of antidepressant drugs for hundreds of victims of depression should not be minimized, their hazards and drawbacks should be carefully evaluated. Natural therapies may accomplish the same goal as these medications, and should be judiciously investigated.

Prozac, the celebrity of antidepressant drugs belongs to the SSRIs. For more detail on Prozac, refer to the following section.

DRUGS USED TO TREAT DEPRESSION

Bicyclic Antidepressant fluoxetine (Prozac)

These are relatively new medications and are currently in widespread use. They function by boosting the production of serotonin in the brain by blocking the re-uptake process. They are known as SSRIs (selective serotonin re-uptake inhibitors). This family of drugs includes Prozac from Eli Lilly, Paxil from Smithkline Beecham and Zoloft from Pfizer.

This class of drugs is considered safer with less side-effects than some of its older counter parts. Drug companies are aggressively promoting them and their market share is growing dramatically. Since they came on the market, more than ten million people worldwide have used them. Close to 1 billion dollars worth of

Prozac was sold last year alone.

Possible side effects include: tremors, nausea, headaches, changes in weight, and a number of other effects. If you take Prozac you may feel agitated, nervous and have trouble sleeping. Nausea and dizziness have also been reported.

Some people taking Prozac believe that it actually made them feel worse. In February of 1990, an article in the *American Journal of Psychiatry* discussed the case of a 40 year old woman who committed suicide while taking Prozac. Doctors at Harvard Medical School's Department of Psychiatry also reported on six people who suddenly became intensely suicidal after 2 to 7 weeks on Prozac.[9] As a result of this study, Harvard psychiatrists have warned that if you take Prozac and feel overly fatigued, restless or oversleep, you may be at a higher risk for an adverse reaction to the drug.

Prozac was introduced by the Eli Lilly Company in 1987. By 1988, Prozac sales were up to $125 million. The following year, sales skyrocketed to $350 million.[10] In its first two years on the market, Americans had spent more on Prozac than on all other twenty antidepressants combined. Projected sales by 1995 were $1 billion. 650,000 prescriptions for Prozac are written each month in this country and that number is expected to reach one million per month in the near future.

Prozac costs approximately $1.50 per pill. If you take Prozac, you can expect to pay between $50 and $200 for treatment depending on your individual dosage. These incredible Prozac statistics dramatically illustrate the magnitude of depressive illness and other related disorders in this country. What's even more distressing, is that even huge numbers like these only tell part of the story. Clearly, depression is a modern day epidemic and its victims are flocking to their doctors for help.

One of the reasons that Prozac has become so popular is that unlike so many other antidepressants, you're not supposed to become heavier, it usually causes weight loss rather than weight gain. If you talk to some women who have taken Prozac, many of them will agree that initially they lost weight, however, after prolonged use, they eventually gained weight and became heavier than when they started. This particular effect is especially troubling and rarely discussed by physicians. These women don't care what side-effect information says about weight loss. The simple fact is that many of them became heavier. One theory suggests that the "I don't care anymore about anything" attitude which Prozac prompts in some of its users created undisciplined eating. As a result of this abnormal nonchalance, eating habits became lax and the motivation to exercise diminished.

Prozac can also have mild stimulant effect which may actually serve to energize some people. Prozac is not only used for depression. It is now commonly prescribed for eating disorders, obsessive-compulsive disorder, and obesity. Its treatment possibilities include: alcoholism, diabetes control, PMS, nicotine withdrawal and drug addiction.[11]

You're probably aware that Prozac has been the subject of considerable controversy and has been implicated in a number of suicides and other examples of erratic behavior. The FDA has determined that Prozac is safe and can be used to treat depression and eating disorders. It's always prudent, concerning any drug that hits the market to investigate side-effects for yourself. If your are considering Prozac or any other antidepressant drug, talk to people who take it and do your homework. Blind assumption that the FDA is omniscient about these matters is foolhardy, to say the least.

The debate surrounding SSRI drugs such as Prozac, Paxil, Zoloft, Lovan and Luvox is that while they raise the level of a certain type of serotonin, they lower another. There is also concern that these drugs act as nervous system stimulants, which can result in altering one's perception of reality and impairing judgement. Despite the conflict enveloping Prozac, many doctors stand by it as a highly effective drug in treating depression.

NOTE: Zoloft, Paxil, Lovan and Luvox are analogues to Prozac. This class of drugs is designed to raise brain levels of serotonin by inhibiting the process of serotonin re-uptake, thereby keeping levels elevated in brain cells. This process prevents serotonin from going into the blood stream. As mentioned earlier, some experts are concerned with this unnatural build up of serotonin in the brain. They warn against a hormonal cascade effect which can, in some individuals, prompt bizarre or destructive behavior.[12]

Tricyclic Antidepressants (TCA'S)

> amitriptyline (Ametril, Elavil, Endep)
> amoxapine (Asendin)
> desipramine (Norpramin, Pertofrane)
> doxepine (Adapin, Sinequan)
> imipramine (Imavate, Janimine, Presamine, Tofranil)
> nortriptyline (Aventyl, Pamelor)
> protriptyline (Vivactil)

These are considered the drugs that are most commonly prescribed for classical depression. The action of these drugs enhances the potency of neurotransmitters in the brain. This particular class of antidepressants is considered safer than MOA inhibitors, however, like any other drug, they have significant side-effects. Some possible side-effects include: drowsiness, increased appetite and weight gain, dry mouth, blurred vision, constipation increased or decreased blood pressure and urinary retention.

Tetracyclic Antidepressant maprotiline (Ludiomil)

Monoamine Oxidase Inhibitors (MAOI's)
phenelzine (Nardil)
tranylcypromine (Parnate)

MAO inhibitors are believed to indirectly stimulate the production of norepinephrine and serotonin in the brain, eliminating deficiencies which can cause depression to occur. They are stimulating rather than sedating in there overall effect and can also cause insomnia, constipation, dry mouth, difficulty focusing, dizziness, uncoordination and skin rashes.

If you take MAO inhibitor drugs you must not eat certain foods which can initiate a sudden rise in blood pressure. These foods contain tyramine and include: cheese, yogurt, ripe bananas, avocados, raisins, canned figs, meats and yeast extracts, pickled fish, marinated meats, chicken liver and some cough and cold medications.

People taking Nardil, Marplan or Parnate must not take any over-the-counter cold or allergy medications that could contain decongestants. Doing so could drastically elevate blood pressure to life-threatening levels. In addition, consuming chocolate, caffeine and several other drugs may cause an adverse reaction if you're taking MOA inhibitors. MOA inhibitors have enough side-effects that most people who take them have to significantly change their lifestyles.

OTHER DRUGS USED TO TREAT DEPRESSION:

alprazolam (Xanax)
lithium (Eskalith, Lithane, Lithobid, Lithotab)
methylphenidate (Ritalin)
trazodone (Desyrel)

Lithium was originally used to treat manic depression, in which drastic mood swings occur. Lithium intake requires close monitoring, as too much can be highly toxic and cause seizures, coma and in extreme cases, death. Other side-effects include: metallic taste in the mouth, stomach upsets, diarrhea, tremors, vomiting, and urine increase.

50 percent of depressions recur even after drug therapy. In these cases, doctors recommend finding an optimal maintenance dose of what they consider the most effective drug to be continued indefinitely. If you find it acceptable to experiment with serious drugs and their dosages to achieve desired results, you should transfer that same attitude to diet, supplementation, etc. Most of us will endlessly fiddle around with potentially harmful medications and rarely examine the effect of vitamins etc. The trial and error method used by doctors to find the right mix should be utilized for natural alternatives as well.

It's not unusual for doctors to use tranquilizers or sedating drugs to treat some of the symptoms that accompany depression, such as insomnia. Librium, Valium, and Ativan are common choices. The *American Journal of Psychiatry* reveals that tranquilizers were the sole medicaiton used in 643 people surveyed who were being treated in outpatient facilities for depression by psychiatrists.[13] These are addictive drugs which may only make matters worse in the long run. Becoming dependent on sleeping pills only further aggravates mood disorders. Sleeping pills do not provide natural, restful sleep, and tranquilizers rarely cure anything, they just suppress symptoms.

There is a growing consensus in this country that drugs are taken too freely and prescribed too easily. Because medicine cabinets everywhere are loaded with all sorts of prescription bottles, the risk of drug abuse is high. Undoubtedly, Americans of all ages are using drugs in greater numbers that ever before and pharmacologic agents designed to elevate moods are one of the most utilized chemicals. The danger here is that frequently, we become dependent on these drugs and may have to increase dosages to receive the result we desire. In some cases, prolonged or habitual users of drugs can develope suicidal tendencies.

CAN NATURAL THERAPIES ACCOMPLISH THE SAME END AS DRUGS?

We've established the fact that most antidepressants are designed to elevate levels of specific brain neurotransmitters. Clearly, if this same effect can be obtained through natural means, side-effects would be minimal. FACT: certain naturally occurring substances can stimulate the same process in the brain which is affected by antidepressant drugs.

It should be stressed at this point, however, that for some people who become profoundly depressed, antidepressant drugs can be potential life-savers. It is the purpose of this book to educate its readers on the value of natural therapies in the treatment of depression. Ideally, all of us would like to do without drugs. It should be realized, however, that in some severe cases of depression, pharmaceuticals may be the only effective means of control. Find out.

Keep in mind that certain natural substances such as amino acids, vitamins, enzymes and minerals can act as precursors to the formation of the brain amines in question and unlike antidepressant drugs, are safer. The bottom line is that there are natural methods available which can create the same desired results as pharmaceutical drugs in the treatment of depression.

Professor Linus Pauling, who has won the Nobel Prize twice for his work coined the term "orthomolecular" psychiatry. This refers to the treatment of mental disease by providing the most optimal molecular environment for the mind through certain concentrations of substances normally present in the body.[14]

The use of these naturally occurring compounds is usually considered much safer than drug therapy. There are countless accounts of people who have died or been injured by medicinal drugs. Dying from a nutrient overdose is extremely rare. Dr. Zoltan P. Rona M.D. points out that there have never been a death as a result of any supplemented vitamin or mineral. By contrast, he emphasizes that something as commonly used as the birth-control pill has 200 known and potentially dangerous side-effects.[15]

Psychiatrists are typically skeptical of the orthomolecular approach to treating any mental disorder. Dr. Pauling firmly believes that nutrition is crucial to the treatment of any mental disorder. He openly condemns the medical establishment's bias against vitamin therapy for mood disorders and points out that various studies conclusively demonstrate that people suffering from schizophrenia absolutely benefited by improving their nutritional status. By taking optimum amounts of niacin, ascorbic acid, thiamine, pyridoxine and other nutrients, their mental outlook improved.

He states: "In 1970 I was walking along Main Street in the small town of Cambria, on the coast of California, when a passing car stopped and the driver got out and ran back to me. She said, `Dr. Pauling, I owe my life to you. I am twenty-six years old. Two years age I was contemplating suicide. I had suffered miserably from schizophrenia for six years. Then I learned about vitamins when someone told me about your paper on orthomolecular psychiatry. The vitamins have saved my life.'"[16]

Unfortunately, in their zeal to protect us from quackery, medical doctors have a tendency to throw the baby out with the bathwater. There is plenty of good scientific evidence that using vitamins and amino acids can successfully treat behavioral disorders, schizophrenia and depression among others. Sadly enough, the immovability of some health care professionals concerning this subject can create a great deal of prejudice and a lack of objectivity.

Consequently, a valuable tool in the treatment of psychological disorders may have been dismissed as worthless. The story is always the same...RDA requirements provide our bodies with all the nutrients we need. If you are eating a balanced diet, you don't need all these supplemental pills.

So, when it comes to getting enough nutrients either to maintain health or treat disease, amounts are determined by preset RDA requirements. RDA requirements set by the government give us the minimum daily allowance of vitamins and mineral necessary to prevent illnesses caused by deficiencies, but do not necessarily refer to dosages needed to maintain optimal health.

While it is fine to presume that food should supply us with all the nutrients we need, it is foolhardy to believe that our diets are all that nutritious. The average American diet is commonly lacking in the B-vitamins, folic acid, Vitamin E, Vitamin C and iron. Ideally, if we routinely consumed a diet comprised of unrefined, unprocessed natural foods, our nutritional needs would be met. Unfortunately, The American diet is typically high in fat, low in complex carbohydrates and fiber, and lacks vitamin C and B-complex.

A number of dietary deficiencies can result in lowered levels of the brain amines needed to maintain a healthy, optimistic mental attitude. Amino acids and vitamins have a direct impact on how we behave and whether we feel like whistling or withdrawing. Prescription drugs treat depression by raising the quantity of certain brain amines. This same end can be accomplished through benign, natural therapies.

There are two different ways to naturally increase the level of certain brain amines or neurotransmitters in the brain. One method is referred to as precursor therapy. A precursor defines a molecule that is converted into a compound such as serotonin of norepinephrine by an particular enzyme. These precursors are normally present in the diet. For example, as discussed earlier, serotonin and norepinephrine are synthesized from the amino acids tryptophan and tyrosine respectively. It makes good sense to assume that the therapeutic use of these amino acids in treating depression is a valid one. Precursor therapy may provide a much safer and effective alternative to increasing these target brain chemicals than standard drug therapy.

The second method involving an orthomolecular treatment for depression raises brain amine levels through cofactor or coenzyme therapy. A cofactor is a compound, (frequently a vitamin) which allows an enzyme to perform its designated chemical function. Vitamin B-6 is the cofactor necessary for the conversion of tryptophan to serotonin and tyrosine to norepinephrine. Obviously, a lack of vitamin B-6 could cause depression by inhibiting the synthesis of brain amines.

By the same token, using Vitamin B-6 in therapeutic doses may effectively treat existing depression by raising the level of these brain chemicals. Dr. Alan Gaby, M.D. states that it is a well documented fact that large doses of B-6 not only raise blood serotonin levels in hyperactive children but can also curb their symptoms.[17]

While using vitamins and other supplements alone may not be the sole answer to treating depression, doctors need to acknowledge the potential value of natural therapies and even more importantly, they need to know when to use them.

FOODS AND MOODS

"A light supper, a good night's sleep and a fine morning have often made a hero of the same man, who by indigestion, a restless night and a rainy morning, would have proved a coward."

The Earl of Chesterfield

Ironically, in some cases of depression, what's eating at you may be the direct result of what you're eating. Brain Weiss, in the December, 1974 issue of *Psychology Today*, states: "'You are what you eat' may turn out to be as true behaviorally as it is bodily. What you are eating may also be what is eating you, and the relation between a six o'clock dinner and a seven o'clock diatribe may be more causal than casual."

What this author is saying is that amino acids which comprise proteins, which compose brain chemicals, which determine mood are all derived from what we choose to eat. The article goes on to stress: "The production of neurochemicals in the brain was once thought to be insulated from the meal-to-meal vagaries of amino acid intake. Recent research, however, concludes that what you eat is what you get...and perhaps how you act."

Most of us are familiar with the link between vitamin C and scurvy, iodine and goiter, calcium and osteoporosis, iron and anemia, rice and beri beri. What we're not familiar with is research that demonstrates the connection between nutrition and behavior, or nutrition and mood disorders.

If you don't believe that things like hunger and what you choose to satisfy that hunger with can affect how you behave, think again. It's a scientific fact that hunger can not only cause physical changes in the body, but emotional ones as well. How many times have you felt grumpy because you've skipped a meal or gone on a carbohydrate restricted diet? Now, what you eat to quell that hunger can set up a complex series of biochemical events that can determine how you'll feel later on, not just physically, but emotionally as well.

A mood change is often our first indication that something is out of kilter with our physiological systems. Scientists at MIT have found that the availability of two amino acids, (tyrosine and tryptophan) in the brain plays a very important role in determining the rate in which four neurotransmitters are produced. Within one hour after a meal, the levels of these brain chemicals begin to change as the amounts of tyrosine and tryptophan fluctuate.

TYPICAL AMERICAN EATING HABITS

If you feel depressed with no apparent reason, what you eat may play a profound causal role. The reverse of this statement is also true; if you are depressed, you probably eat poorly, thereby perpetrating your low mood. You might think you can get away with eating poorly. Be assured that, to the contrary, if you neglect you dietary health, you'll eventually have to pay the piper in one respect or another.

The sad fact is that most depressed people, or undepressed people for that matter, don't eat well. How many of us gulp down a bowl of sugary cereal or a sweet roll for breakfast, washed down with one or more cups of coffee, have a caffeine drink and french fries for lunch and then order a pizza for dinner? An individual who consumes three cups of coffee, a chocolate candy bar, a cola drink and two headache pills ingests around 400 milligrams of caffeine in one day, an amount which can cause severe mental and emotional disturbances.[18]

Our society is becoming so caffeine dependent that psychiatrists have coined a new phrase for their diagnostic manual called "caffeinism." Our obsession with caffeine consumption has made it the most widely used drug in the world. Cola drinks are the most popular beverage in this country and are routinely used by children as well. Festive and fun Coke and Pepsi commercials fail to tell us that caffeine is a strong and addictive drug.

We won't go into all the physiological affects of caffeine at this point. It should suffice to know that caffeine is a mental stimulant that affects the way your brain and nervous system work. From an emotional standpoint, an excess of caffeine can result in insomnia, anxiety, panic attacks, delirium, and wild mood fluctuations.

Because caffeine initially stimulates the release of norepinephrine, you may experience a temporary lift from your cup of coffee or big gulp. In time, if you consistently use caffeine, brain amine supplies can become depleted and feelings of nervousness and fatigue may occur.

Caffeine can also inhibit your body's ability to absorb vitamin B-1 and cause you to lose magnesium. The link between magnesium and mood swings is discussed in the section on vitamins and minerals. Some people are easily cured of a whole host of mental and physical symptoms just by eliminating all caffeine and adding a good daily supply of B-vitamins. These people are usually oblivious to the enormous amounts of caffeine they consume.

For years, professionals in the health and nutrition field have warned against the side-effects of caffeine. Only recently, has the scientific community taken notice. Caffeine emphasizes the fact that what we consume does affect how we behave. See the section on Unrecognized Causes of Depression for more information on caffeine.

The field of nutrition and its relationship to the treatment of disease has been notorious for spawning conflicting theories and controversial claims. Today, more than ever before, medical doctors are finally officially advocating what health and nutrition specialists have been saying for years. Ancient physicians knew that food could either agitate or calm the mind. Today, modern medicine needs to re-learn what has been known all along; that diet affects individual behavior.

Scientific evidence has now vindicated what were considered several nutritional hoaxes of the past: that less fat and sugar more fiber, fresh vegetables, whole grains dramatically lowers the risk for some forms of cancer, diabetes, heart disease, and colon disorders. Interestingly, according to a new study reported in the November, 1992 *Annals of Internal Medicine*, when people lowered their cholesterol over a five-year study period, they also experienced a reduction in depression and hostility.

Using food to treat or prevent disease is nothing new. Johns Hopkins University uses a ketogenic diet to treat pediatric epilepsy and the calcium/osteoporosis connection is widely advocated among today's doctors. To assume that future research will support additional correlations made between diet and mental health is probable, to say the least. Unfortunately, because natural treatments and diets are not patentable, you may not find out about these alternatives unless you investigate for yourself. The ketogenic diet for children with epilepsy has been around for decades. Sadly enough, only a very small percentage of parents were aware of the diet's existence. As soon as their children experienced their first seizure, they were immediately put on anticonvulsant drugs and told to get on with their lives. Something as simple as producing ketones in the body, which is what the ketogenic diet does can decrease seizures and even cure a significant number of children who suffer from epilepsy. Again, food profoundly affects brain function. Who knew?

Have you ever noticed that after you eat certain foods, you feel like your mood and energy levels literally crash? Some people feel sudden elation or depression within a few hours of ingesting certain foods or beverages. Dr. Morris Lipton of the University of North Carolina and chairman of the first federally funded conference on nutrition says that the link between food and mood is undeniable.[19]

DIET...A CAUSE OF DEPRESSION?

It is the opinion of several nutritionists and orthomolecular psychiatrists, who emphasize the role of nutrition for the treatment of mental disorders that diet is the most frequent cause of depression. Dr. Harvey M. Ross M.D. believes that many psychiatrists are experiencing a loss of esteem due to their refusal to investigate the value of nutritive therapy for mental disorders. He stresses that this lack of objectivity has resulted in the dismissal of a very valuable psychiatric tool.[20] The time has come for anyone who seeks professional treatment for, not only depression, but any other physical or mental disorder to educate themselves on nutritive options to treating disease.

Interestingly, a deficiency of just about any nutrient can result in depression. If you eat poorly for an extended period of time, you inadvertently effect brain neurotransmitters. Even rats who were put on nutritionally deficient diets became lethargic, indifferent and withdrawn. A later section on vitamins discusses which nutrients are particularly relevant to mood disorders.

Most of us would agree that Americans eat way too much junk

food and snack on sweet, empty, calorie laden foods. What we call food today some times stretches the imagination. Michael Jacobson, in the April, 1975 edition of *Smithsonian* states:

"The United States, not surprisingly, has been the leader in the genetic engineering of food crops and in the laboratory creation of new foods. Benjamin Franklin and Abraham Lincoln, if they could visit us, would probably have some difficulty distinguishing between a toy store and a supermarket. They would not even recognize as foods such products as artificial whipped cream in its pressurized can, or some breakfast 'cereals' that are almost half sugar and bear little resemblance to cereal grains...Many of the new foods do save us time and trouble, but they are often costly, in terms of both dollars and, ultimately, health."

The impact of that way we eat in this country on mental health and behavior remains virtually unexplored. In other words, we have barely scratched the surface when it comes to understanding how our diet effects our brain.

Brain chemicals, like other cellular substances are controlled to a great extent by diet and genetic predispositions. Researchers at the Massachusetts Institute of Technology have discovered that the chemistry of the brain and its various functions are greatly effected by what we choose to eat. According to Dr. Judith Wurtman, who has done extensive research in this field, there are three groups of foods that cause quick and dramatic changes in brain activity:

- Carbohydrates (whole grains, vegetables, sugars) which promote calm, reduce anxiety and stress and help to focus the mind
- Proteins (animal foods, legumes) which help to promote the stimulation of the brain and produce energy.
- Caffeine, which also acts as a brain stimulant and a temporary energy source.[21]

It is generally accepted that heighted levels of awareness occur when levels of dopamine or norepinephrine rise by eating protein meals that contain essential fatty acids and some carbohydrates. For some people, eating carbohydrates alone, which promotes serotonin production, results in easing tension and creating a sensation of calm.

Most people who go on a good, nutritious diet that eliminates caffeine, fatty, junk foods, white flours, sugar etc. find that they receive the unexpected benefit of a hard-to-describe feeling of well-being. Eating whole grains and plenty of fresh raw fruits and vegetables can create a newfound feeling of focus and emotional stability. Foods that are full of vitamin B-complex can actually help to pacify the nervous system. While scientific skeptics may scoff, there is no question that what we eat can determine whether we have a good sense of self or one that is anxious and disturbed.

Personally speaking, I have found that after eating a diet that was full of rich, fatty, sugary foods for an extended period of time, not only do I feel physically lousy, but I feel emotionally off as well. The human body automatically reacts to what is naturally good or bad for it. If you are in tune with yourself, you can see a significant difference when diet is modified. It is virtually impossible to separate the physical from the mental, spiritual or emotional self. All facets of our being are affected by our individual lifestyles. To assume that depression may be a by-product of that lifestyle is plausible, to say the least.

The fact remains that brain chemicals or amines can be manufactured by utilizing and increasing the amounts of certain vitamins, minerals and amino acids readily available in most health food stores. The key lies is seeing for yourself. The scientific data is conclusive. What we ingest has a definite bearing on our mental outlook as well as our physical status.

Why were there less depressed people among our pioneer ancestors? Over the last thirty years, modern technology has changed what we eat and the way we eat it. We now routinely consume new crop varieties which have been genetically engineered, hormonally fattened beef and poultry, foods that have undergone a number of high-tech processing techniques, and a wide variety of food additives and preservatives.

Foods are no longer eaten in season as in past generations. Fruits and vegetables are shipped transcontinentally and are often packed in dry ice or refrigerated for extended periods of time. In addition, new foods have been created and synthetic food substitutes like Nutra-Sweet and synthetic fats are rapidly dominating commercially packaged foods. Most breakfast cereals hardly resemble the whole grains our grandparents would have eaten for breakfast, and millions of gallons of sugary or artificially sweetened soda pop are consumed annually.

Since the 1940's, our systems have been exposed to thousands of new chemicals which have found their way into not only our foods, but our air and water as well. RDA (recommended daily allowances) of vitamins and minerals were never set up to deal with the mental and physical stressors that typify our environment.

There can be no question that all of these nutritional alterations play a significant role in the incidence of mental illness and mood disorders that currently afflict our generation. This doesn't imply that other factors aren't involved. Certain circumstances can trigger brain amine imbalances, such as the loss of a job, or even the birth of a baby. It stands to reason that if depression can be induced by a malfunction of the brain's biochemistry, whatever the source, then it should respond to nutritional modifications. Moreover, some cases of depression may be caused by the actual lack of certain nutrients or the misuse of others.

Nutrition can be the single most important therapy in fighting certain types of depression. Dr. Ross claims that the investigation of diet can be one of the most important measures taken in determining how to treat depression and is, unfortunately, also one of the most overlooked treatments. He mentions the role of low blood sugar, or hypoglycemia, which is determined by our intake of carbohydrates as a major factor to be considered.

_____ SUGAR AND MOOD SWINGS

"If God meant us to eat sugar, he wouldn't have invented dentists."

Ralph Nader

The average American eats over 125 pounds of white sugar every year. It has been estimated, that sugar makes up 25 percent of our daily calorie intake, with soda pop supplying the majority of that intake. Desserts and sugar-laden snacks constantly tempt us and our taste for rich desserts escalates as we consume more and more. Americans eat an average of 15 quarts of ice cream per person per year. We have become a sugar obsessed people and the ramifications of this kind of extreme consumption would undoubtedly fill volumes.

The facts are blatant, the amount of sugar we consume as a country has to have a profound effect on both our physical and mental well being. Sugar is a powerful substance which can have drug-like effects and is considered addictive by a number of nutritional experts. Our diets are loaded with sugar, hidden or added from our first bowl of sugared cold cereal, to our daily big gulp, to our typical consumption of chips, candy bars and pastries.

In excess amounts, sugar can be toxic. Sufficient amounts of B-vitamins are actually required to metabolize and detoxify sugar in our bodies. When you overload your body with sugar you can inhibit the assimilation of nutrients from other foods. In other words, our bodies were not designed to cope with the high quantity of sugar we routinely ingest. Too much sugar can generate a type of nutrient malnutrition which, according to a number of experts, can affect the way we behave. In addition, too much sugar can predispose us to yeast infections, aggravate some types of arthritis and asthma, cause tooth decay and may elevate the level of our blood lipids.

WHY DO WE CRAVE WHAT'S SO BAD FOR US?

Considering these sobering facts, why do we eat so much sugar? It's hard to ignore a bad sweet tooth and the question remains: if its so bad for you, why do we find ourselves intensely craving sugar? Sugar gives us a quick infusion of energy. Naturally, we need carbohydrates to survive. The notion, however, that in the twentieth century we would have instant access to unlimited amounts of sugar was unanticipated by our physiology. The human body was not set up to process such enormous quantities of sugar.

Our extraordinary craving form sugar stems from a complex mix of physiological and psychological components. Even the most brilliant scientists fail to totally comprehend this intriguing chemical dependence which, for the most part, hurts our health. Having a sweet tooth can contribute to PMS, osteoporosis, coronary artery disease, diabetes, obesity and depression. The added subconscious suggestion that sweets can serve as a reward for good behavior compounds the problem further. Desserts are commonly viewed as the way we pat ourselves on the back.

Ironically, most of our children don't think of sugary foods as "treats" anymore. Some subsist on them. Twenty years ago, candy was only available to most American children at Christmastime, or during Halloween. A fresh orange in the Christmas stocking was considered a wonderful and sweet delicacy.

Today, our homes, schools and workplaces are teeming with candy, cookies, cakes, highly sweetened cold cereal, pop etc. What is so insidious about consuming sugar is that the more you eat, the more you want. Unbeknownst to most of us, eating sugar in these unnatural amounts can also affect the way we view ourselves and the world, whether we're agreeable or cantankerous. Here lies the ultimate biological paradox. Frequently, we crave the very substances that not only is hard for our physiology to tolerate but can make us act "intolerable" as well.

Have you ever been around someone who is prone to mood swings characterized by violent verbal attacks and sudden irritability. No one just goes on an unprovoked rampage out of the blue. This type of volatile behavior is typical of some people who crave sugar, eat it and then experience subsequent behavioral symptoms. Erratic mood swings can be linked to dramatic drops in blood sugar levels referred to as hypoglycemia, which is discussed in a later section of this chapter. What is really interesting is that craving sugar to begin with, may be related to drops in brain amine levels which can make you feel lethargic and "low." There go those brain amines again.

SEROTONIN LEVELS AND CARBOHYDRATE CRAVINGS

If you find yourself strongly craving snacks like cookies or chips on a consistent basis and you suffer from depression, your mood fluctuations may be related to serotonin levels which can be effected by the presence of sugar in the blood stream. The Wurtman Study revealed that people who crave carbohydrates showed a high susceptibility to clinical depression.[22] In other words, if you have a tendency to crave carbohydrate snacks, you may not be eating just to satisfy hunger. Do you eat just one or two cookies if you occasionally crave something sweet? If you find yourself eating cookie after cookie or consuming half a bag of chips at one sitting, you may be a victim of a carbohydrate related mood disorder.

When people who typically snacked this way were asked why they constantly ate foods they knew would create weight problems, they responded that they ate to combat tension, feelings of anxiety or mental fatigue. The result of eating several cookies or potato chips was the creation of a feeling of calmness and well-being. Further research at MIT has shown that some obese people use sugar or carbohydrates as a type of sedative to maintain this sense of well-being. When their sugar levels drop, their feelings of anxiety return.[23]

An additional study done at MIT administered psychological tests to 46 volunteers before and after they ate a meal rich in carbohydrates. Those who were considered habitual carbohydrate cravers were shown to be significantly less depressed after ingesting the food. On the other hand, non-cravers became tired and sleepy.[24]

What is significant about these findings is that appetite fluctuations may be motivated by mood disorders. This implies that for some people, food cravings are the body's way of trying to elevate certain neurotransmitters in the brain that create sensations of security and contentment. In so doing, some people find themselves continually craving and snacking, a phenomenon which is not always related to true hunger. Frequently, people who fall into this category will gain weight due to the caloric nature of most carbohydrate snacks, which only further serves to decrease their feelings of self-worth.

The brain chemical involved here is called serotonin, which is a derivative of tryptophan, an amino acid. The rate in which this amino acid is converted to serotonin depends on the amount of carbohydrates consumed. Blood levels of tryptophan increase when carbohydrates are eaten. Tryptophan crosses the blood-brain barrier and is converted into serotonin. The rate of this conversion is dependent on the proportion of carbohydrates eaten. Carbohydrates stimulate the production of insulin which permits the uptake of most amino acids into cells. What is important to realize here is that studies like this indicate that when brain levels of serotonin decrease, some people begin to crave carbohydrates.[25]

The study also points out that in some people who have trouble with mood swings or even PMS, the brain fails to respond as it should when starchy snacks are eaten, therefore the craving persists and overeating occurs. More importantly, if you seek medical treatment for your depression and you are put on an antidepressant that is designed to block serotonin transmission in the brain, or one that interacts with brain chemicals other than serotonin, carbohydrate cravings will increase and weight gain will occur.

The link with these findings and people who suffer from low blood sugar, which causes an intense craving for carbohydrates is interesting to say the least. If the carbohydrates craved were complex carbohydrates, the outcome may be somewhat different. It is the over-consumption of what has been referred to as "naked" carbohydrates in the form of white sugar and white flour that seem particularly detrimental to both our physical and mental health.

THE PERILS OF SUGAR

Eating too much sugar not only depletes our bodies of vitamin B, which is crucial to maintaining a healthy a mental outlook, it can also contribute to amino acid depletion, which has a direct influence on mood. Tryptophan and phenylalanine have to compete with sugar for absorption in the intestines. For this reason, nutritionists have long advised against eating protein and sugar at the same time. To make matters worse, eating excess sugar can weaken and compromise our immune systems by lowering white blood cell counts which makes us susceptible to colds and other infections and diseases. Like a narcotic, taking sugar initially makes us feel better, but its "high" comes with an exorbitant cost to our health.

Some experts believe that sugar is physically addictive. In the book *Sugar Blues,* William Dufty writes, "The difference between sugar addiction and narcotic addiction is largely one of degree." Perhaps it would be more accurate to refer to sugar as a substance that has a drug-like affect on the body. In and of itself, a moderate amount of sugar consumed now and then may be perfectly harmless to most people. The potential problem, however, with eating a little sugar is that because of its easy access, over-indulging occurs all to often.

I know that if I eat a lot of sweets over the holidays, I find it very difficult to taper off afterwards. Eating sweets creates the craving for more sweets. January is particularly bad because the residual effects of December feasting are still operational. The worst part is if you abruptly cut off your sweet supply, you can feel fatigued, irritable, headachy and depressed. It is this abnormal dependence that so many of us have on sugar that is believed to spawn a number of disorders. In our discussion of depression, hypoglycemia is perhaps the most significant of these.

——— HYPOGLYCEMIA AND DEPRESSION

"Beware of poisons dressed in sweet's clothing"
Anonymous

It is hard to image the havoc that a benign looking substance like sugar can wreak. When it comes to unexplained depression, the role of sugar can be explosive to say the least. The brain is extremely depended on glucose or blood sugar as it prime energy source. A sudden drop in glucose levels can result in the release of hormone, designed to bring that level up again. For some of us, eating sugar causes an exaggeration of this biochemical response. Consequently, we experience of number of undesirable side-effects.

What's distressing is that you may be one of these people and not even know it. As a result, you continue eating a diet high in the very substance that may be compromising the quality of your life. Simply put, mental health and emotional behavior are both intimately linked with blood sugar levels, a factor which has been badly overlooked by conventional medicine.

We've already established the sad fact that most of us subsist on a diet comprised of sugar, white flour, alcohol and other refined "foods." These substances are, in truth, nutritionally worthless and can, in fact, deplete our bodies of valuable nutrients. The human body was not meant to ingest the abnormally high quantities of sugar most of us eat each and every day.

For some of us, who are sugar sensitive, eating excess amounts of sugar can propel us into dramatic mood swings not to mention a whole host of other undesirable symptoms. For all the visits, medical testing, and drug and psychotherapy you might have tried, your depression could be caused and sustained by drops in blood sugar levels.

Before you try to design a natural treatment program for your depression, make sure that your problem doesn't stem from low blood sugar commonly referred to as "sugar blues" or hypoglycemia. This term is defined as a condition of abnormal sugar metabolism which results in abnormally low levels of blood sugar. Eating too much sugar or refined carbohydrates can bring about hypoglycemic reactions in some individuals. In addition, be aware of the fact that some medications, including Prozac can make you prone to drops in blood sugar levels.

HYPOGLYCEMIA: A FAD DISEASE?

Much controversy has surrounded hypoglycemia within the medical establishment. Unfortunately, the majority of physicians shake their heads when you mention the term hypoglycemia. Most doctors believe that this condition is extremely rare or is directly related to diabetics who may get too much insulin. They consider it a "fad" disease which has no physiological basis. Because hypoglycemia is rarely understood by the medical community, it is often brushed off as a bogus malady. One reason for this denial is the inadequacies of the 5-hour glucose tolerance test (GTT) as an effective diagnostic tool.

In reality, hypoglycemia is believed to cause a great deal of misery. Moreover, new studies are revealing that certain psychological disorders are directly linked with disturbed glucose utilization in brain cells. One study, in particular, showed that depressed people have overall lower glucose metabolism which is most concentrated in the front and left sections of the brain.[26]

The truth is that many perfectly normal, otherwise healthy people experience dramatic swings in their blood sugar levels. Low blood sugar, in fact, can initiate a number of troublesome symptoms, including depression. I can honestly tell you that if eat a bowl of highly sugared cold cereal like Captain Crunch, I go into some serious tremors approximately two hours later. This type of artificial food is ultra-refined. It shoots your blood sugar level up so high, so fast that the pancreas tries to compensate with a large secretion of insulin that ends up taking blood sugar levels to extreme lows. Consequently, you can experience some pretty frightening symptoms, which I almost always do.

What's happening is this: if too much insulin is secreted in order to compensate for high blood sugar, which results from eating an excess of carbohydrates, blood sugar drops. As a result, glucagon, cortisol and adrenalin are poured out into the system to help raise blood sugar back to acceptable levels. This can inadvertently result in the secretion of more insulin to bring it back down and the vicious cycle goes on. Achieving proper blood sugar balance is tricky business and eating the wrong things can throw the system into extreme responses.

Did you know that high insulin secretion can cause substantial changes in brain chemistry? Are you aware of the fact that ingesting caffeine can adversely affect blood sugar levels. Eating sugary foods can propel the pancreas, pituitary, and adrenal glands into a highly complex chemical reaction based on a feedback loop. The irony of this hypoglycemic cycle is that when blood sugar drops, we run for more sugar and we, ourselves, perpetrate the disorder.

Hypoglycemia is not a new disease. It's a forgotten or denied disease. Dr. Seal Harris actually received an award by the American Medical Association for developing a high-protein, low sugar diet with frequent meals to help people who experienced lowered blood sugar after eating sugar.[27] Unfortunately, most doctors are reluctant to recognize the fact that depression might be the result of lowered blood glucose.

In some circles, hypoglycemia is considered the most common cause of depression. In a study of 500 people with hypoglycemia, 75% were found to be suffering from significant depression.[28] Dr. Harvey Ross, M.D. believes that hypoglycemia is so prevalent that it is mandatory to consider the possibility of this disorder whenever a patient complains of depression. Something as benign and seemingly harmless as sugar can play the role of a menacing mood disrupter.

Ironically, if you suffer from low blood sugar, the more depressed you are, the more you crave sugar. Joan Davidson puts it this way..."Sugar addiction is a common factor in hypoglycemia; most people who suffer from this disease have a severe sweet tooth. They crave sugar as an upper because it increases their blood sugar levels and make them feel less lethargic."[29]

Several open-minded physicians who encounter people complaining of depression will check to see if hypoglycemia is a factor. A glucose tolerance test will be administered. Keep in mind that this test is not always accurate. Dr. David R. Hawkins, medical director of the North Nassau Mental Health Center has performed five-hour glucose tests which were perfectly normal for the first three hours and then showed a dramatic drop during the fourth hour. Dr. Ross points out that 90 percent of treatable hypoglycemia can be missed when physicians assess the results from a strict predetermined point that has been designated as normal.[30]

He stresses that recently research has suggested that 50mg.% is too high a reading. He points out that determining at what level symptoms of hypoglycemia will occur is extremely difficult and varies with each individual. What is normal for one person, may not be for another. He goes on to say that sometimes he has seen test results that were normal, however, the patient felt awful during and after the test and showed typical symptoms of hypoglycemia. He cautions against relying solely on test numbers.

Sadly, there are numerous people who struggle with low-blood sugar depression for years, barely functioning. A simple switch from a diet high in refined carbohydrates to one comprised of protein and some complex carbohydrates could have meant the difference between a dysfunctional life and a rich one. People who have had hypoglycemic mood disorders frequently comment that they feel as if they have gotten off of an emotional seesaw after going on a good nutritious diet which is supplemented with vitamin and minerals.

One such person described himself as "incredibly depressed." He referred to himself as a zombie who frequently missed work and had great difficulty just dragging himself out of bed in the morning. Morning for him meant feeling lousy. He felt exhausted, woke up with a headache and felt nauseated. He comments, "At least I know my nausea and headache aren't due to pregnancy. But the bad side is that what I've got has lasted more than six months."[31]

This man was subsequently tested for glucose intolerance and related to his present physician that he suspected he had hypoglycemia, but had received no support from his previous encounters with doctors. Not one of these doctors had asked him about his dietary habits, and certainly, none of them suggested modifying his diet or using vitamin supplements. In questioning this man, it was discovered that he, like so many other Americans, had practically lived on Coke and Candy bars. These two popular dietary foods have been referred to by some doctors as the "nutritional precursors of depression."[32] Likewise, the caffeine and chocolate duo should be viewed in the same way.

This person was subsequently placed on a low carbohydrate diet using millet and low fat meat that was supplemented with vitamin B-6, vitamin B-12, folic acids, tryptophan and pantothenic acid. His recovery was not immediate and his doctor adjusted his vitamin and amino acid levels. Within a month, he felt one-hundred percent better. His depression was gone.

DO YOU HAVE HYPOGLYCEMIA?

Examining your eating habits; what you eat and when you eat it, and what happens during the following hours may be more informative than any diagnostic lab test. Anyone who feels depressed in combination with crying spells, anxiety, headaches or apprehension should suspect low blood sugar levels. In addition, you need to examine your genetic history. Hypoglycemia runs in families.

Some studies have shown that up to 77% of people who experience low blood sugar suffer from depression.[33] Unquestionably, people who suffer from low blood sugar or hypoglycemia are strongly predisposed to depression. Oscar Janiger M.D. in his book, *A Different Kind of Healing* talks about one of his patients who had been treated for depression with drugs and psychotherapy for ten years.

After reading a magazine article she announced to him that she had been misdiagnosed and really should have been treated for low blood sugar. Naturally, Dr. Janiger was skeptical, to say the least, but reluctantly administered a blood glucose test which revealed that she did indeed suffer from hypoglycemia. Anyone who consistently battles depression that cannot be connected with any other factors should investigate the possibility that they have low blood sugar.

One Colorado internist comments:

"People who are chronically stressed and are on a roller coaster of blood sugar going up and down are especially prone to dips in energy at certain times of day. Their adrenals are not functioning optimally, and when they hit a real low point, they want sugar. It usually happens in mid-afternoon when the adrenal glands are at their lowest level of functioning. I have them take glutamine at that point because it helps to regulate the glucose in the brain."[34]

The brain is highly dependent on glucose (blood sugar) for its energy source. When blood sugar levels drop, hormones go into action. It is the release of adrenalin that causes the "sugar shakes" including sweating, tremors, hunger and weakness. These very obvious symptoms usually accompany a sudden and dramatic drop in blood sugar. Keep in mind that if your blood sugar levels decrease gradually, you may not recognize your symptoms as those of hypoglycemia. You may feel dizzy, confused, clouded, and emotionally unstable without any visible tremors.

In cases of depression that were caused by hypoglycemia, low energy levels in the absence of any event that would normally accompany the "blues" are the rule. People who suffer from this kind of depression will often comment that they have a good life and should be happy but they feel downcast and glum. They also routinely mention that to call their erratic behavior abnormal is an understatement.

Anxiety attacks can become a part of hypoglycemic mood swings. Other emotional symptoms of hypoglycemia include apathy, paranoia, phobias, delusions, confusion and severe anxiety. The following symptoms can result from a blood sugar instability or hypoglycemia. Notice how many of the symptoms are the same as those listed for classic depression.

- nervousness
- irritability, outburst, rage
- crying spells
- exhaustion
- faintness, dizziness, tremor, cold sweats, hot flashes
- depression
- vertigo
- drowsiness
- headaches
- intense craving for sweets or uncontrolled appetite
- digestive disturbances
- forgetfulness
- excessive sighing and yawning
- impotence
- moods which fluctuate throughout the day
- insomnia
- anxiety or excessive worrying

- social withdrawal
- mental confusion
- heart palpitations
- muscle pains, leg cramps
- numbness
- indecisiveness
- allergies

Typically, if you suffer from hypoglycemia, you will feel good right after you eat and then your mood and-physical status will deteriorate two to six hours after you eat.

If you suspect that you might suffer from low blood sugar, examine your dietary history carefully. Do your have a family history of diabetes, alcoholism or low blood sugar? Do you crave carbohydrates on a consistent basis? Do you feel terrible both physically and mentally in the morning? If you have several of the symptoms listed above, you may wish to read *Fighting Depression* by Harvey Ross, M.D. who delineates in detail the dietary strategy necessary to control this disorder.

It's wise to remember that a drop in blood sugar can induce mental symptoms which are often confused with depression itself. They include: fatigue, melancholy, irritability, hostility, confusion, paranoia, and anxiety.

TO EAT OR NOT TO EAT...FOOD CHOICES TO PREVENT SUGAR BLUES

In several cases of depression, when foods were eliminated from the diet that cause severe blood sugar swings, patients were able to control their depression even when years of psychotherapy failed them. Sugar and caffeine have been singled out as being the "first to go" when adjusting the diet to alleviate mood swings. Frequently, just the elimination of these two substance from the system can be incredibly beneficial in helping to control and avoid depressed mental states all together. The elimination of foods such as candy, soda pop, doughnuts and other sugary pastries, sugared cold cereals, cookies etc. cannot be over-emphasized. These types of foods quickly raise blood glucose levels and initiate a rush of insulin, which brings those levels way down.

Don't underestimate the emotional ill-effects of caffeine combined with sugar. People with mental or emotional disorders pay a heavy price for using caffeine, especially in the form of coffee. Heavy coffee drinkers consistently score higher on tests for depression and anxiety than other people[35] Coffee contains from 29 to 176 milligrams of caffeine, cola drinks about 40 milligrams and a chocolate bar, approximately 25 milligrams. Even if you eliminate these substances from your diet, watch out for hidden sources of caffeine found in some headache medicines and appetite suppressants.

If you suffer from hypoglycemia, substituting whole grains, fresh vegetables and supplementing the diet with B-vitamins, vitamin C and chromium can, in some cases, eliminate the need for antidepressant or anti-anxiety drugs. Some doctors will recommend a diet that is rich in protein and complex carbohydrates, with the elimination of refined foods and all caffeine. Make a resolve to start eating healthily.

Dr. August F. Daro, an obstetrician/gynecologist in Chicago says, "A lot of depressed people don't eat well... perhaps they'll have a cup of coffee and a sweet roll for breakfast. I make sure they eat three good meals every day. A good diet has to be the foundation of the nutritional treatment of depression."[36]

It is interesting to learn that nocturnal hypoglycemia, which refers to a low night time blood sugar level, can also promote insomnia. As mentioned earlier, when blood sugar drops, adrenaline is released which stimulates the brain and signals to the body that it is time to eat. If you eat a whole grain snack 30 minutes before going to bed, you can avoid this scenario.

Complex carbohydrates that take time to break down can help to sustain normal blood sugar levels throughout the night. In addition, as we have discussed, these types of foods increase serotonin levels in the brain which helps to promote sleep. Whatever you do, don't eat highly refined, sugary snacks before going to bed. Eating foods like a big bowl of sugar frosted flakes before you go to bed is one of the worse things you can do.

It should be realized that when some people stop eating white sugar and refined carbohydrates they may feel worse at first due to the effects of sugar withdrawal. Mood swings may still be a problem. If this is the case, Dr. Ross, suggests eating wholesome snacks that are high in protein or complex carbohydrates every two hours to prevent the blood sugar from dropping. He also recommends adding B-complex vitamins to help boost the function of the nervous system. [37]

In summary then, if you suspect that you are hypoglycemic and suffer from depression emphasize the following foods:

white meats, fish, nuts and seeds, whole grains including whole grain pastas, unsweetened yogurt, vegetable juices and eggs, low carbohydrate vegetables such as celery, beet greens, chives, cucumbers, lettuce, parsley, radishes, asparagus, broccoli, cabbage, cauliflower, mushrooms, onions, peppers, tomatoes, squash, spinach and zucchini.

Fruits should be limited to two servings per day and should be eaten as part of a meal rather than a separate snack. Recommended fruits include:

berries, cantaloupe, coconut, muskmelon, cranberries, casaba melon, and lemons/limes

AVOID:

All processed or enriched foods like white flour or sugar, quick cooking grains, artificial sweeteners, caffeine, alcohol, and high fat, empty calorie foods like doughnuts, pastries, cakes, soda pop etc.

Eat small meals throughout the day supplemented with protein snacks. A snack or mini meal every two hours is recommended. Raw almonds are excellent.

Supplementing any hypoglycemic diet with B-complex vitamins, vitamin E, pantothenic acid, and vitamin C and vitamin E is desireable. Dr. Ross also adds L-glutamine, an amino acid which appears to boost brain nutrition to the mix.

Keep in mind that when you first start to eat this way, you will probably feel lousy. You may feel weak, dizzy, nauseous and get even more depressed. This is particularly true if you have been eating a diet high in white sugar and fat. Give the diet a chance. Your body takes time to adjust and beneficial results won't be seen overnight.

If you persevere and endure, typically the next phase brings a dramatic improvement in feelings of physical well being and mental elevation. You'll still have good days and bad days. In time, you'll notice less variation of mood as your body adjusts and more energy, however, you may still find it difficult to stick to the diet as the cravings for sugar and high carbohydrates may persist. If you continue, within three to five weeks, you should start to notice all kind of good things. You should be able to think better, wake up easier and generally feel good about life. Remember that the nutritional treatment of depression requires the teamwork of a revised diet, boosted by certain supplements, and the accurate evaluation of the biochemical response of each individual. In other words, it takes time to find the winning combinations and doses for each person. Find yourself a doctor who is willing to work with this kind of therapy.

DEPRESSION AND AMINO ACIDS

"Nature never breaks her own laws"
Leonardo da Vinci

Who knows what an amino acid is? Amino acids are nothing more than natural substances which comprise the building blocks of proteins. Amino acids are closely linked with the mind and the emotions in that they are required to manufacture the chemical messengers of the brain, called neurotransmitters. Neurotransmitters are comprised of proteins. In order to transmit nerve impulses effectively, certain levels of these brain chemicals must be available. In the case of depression and other mental conditions, a lack of a particular neurotransmitter seems to be the culprit.

Out of all the natural therapies for depression, amino acids command our attention. Amino acid therapy for mood disorders and other nervous system afflictions promises to become one of the more promising natural treatments for disease. There is significant evidence that using amino acids in therapeutic doses can boost brain levels of specific neurotransmitters requires to prevent the onset of depression.

Amino acids serve in a variety of vital functions in the body. One of the objectives of taking certain free-form amino acids is to initiate the production and concentration of serotonin and norepinephrine, two mood altering brain chemicals, we should all be familiar with by now.

If you think that your diet is good and probably supplies you with plenty of amino acids, you may be surprised to learn that some studies have shown that only 60 percent of people who appear to be in good health have normal levels of all amino acids in their blood.

One explanation for this is the fact that while we may be eating protein, the useability of that protein, may not be ideal. In other words, you can eat a lot of protein foods and be ingesting protein that is inferior in quality. For example, if you eat lots of fish, you may be getting enough useable protein. If your diet is high in dairy products, however, you may assume you're getting plenty of protein, when in fact the availability of that particular kind of protein may be significantly decreased.

AMINO ACIDS AS PRECURSORS TO MOOD INFLUENCING BRAIN CHEMICALS

Because protein is not always assimilated efficiently, you may be deficient in the specific amino acids that are required to produce certain key neurotransmitters that control mood. Norepinephrine, serotonin, dopamine, acetylcholine and histamine are referred to as "precursor" dependent. In other words, their production depends on the availability of precursors or amino acids derived from your diet. Increasing the amount of precursors in the brain to boost the production of these chemicals is dependent on eating specific nutrients that are converted into these key substances.

Because amino acids compete with each other for assimilation and because just eating protein foods does not ensure an increase in these precursors, a deficiency can exist. Taking amino acid supplements creates precursor loading in the brain which diet alone may not provide. Consequently, if this precursor loading is going to work, amino acids must be taken individually as singular free form amino acids and in the proper quantities to enable the chemical process to proceed effectively. Feeling mentally dismal can be the direct result of an insufficiency of these amine precursors which are not being properly utilized or supplied by the diet. In these individuals, precursor loading or amino acid therapy can prove invaluable.

In one of its latest assessments of various alternative therapies, The American Psychiatric Association stated that amino acid therapies may have a great deal to offer in the treatment of psychiatric disease. I would assume that a statement of this caliber which originates from the medical community will have profound future implications for accepted modes of treating behavioral disorders.

Amino acids are much less expensive and have far less side-effects than drugs. Acceptance of this new approach to treating depressive illness is gaining support around the world and is considered a much safer alternative than most mood altering drugs.

Simply stated, brain amines are produced from amino acids. Through the proper supplementation of amino acids, the production of certain brain amines can be stimulated. It is vital to understand, at this point, that if amino acid therapy is to be effective, certain vitamins and minerals must be added to the mix.

TRYPTOPHAN, TYROSINE, AND PHENYLALANINE

L-tyrosine, L-phenylalanine and L-tryptophan are considered the most effective amino acids in treating depression. It is recommended that a qualified physician supervise any amino acid therapy you may wish to try. Certain specifics must be followed in order to ensure the effectiveness of this type of treatment. Amino acids have to be taken at certain times, on an empty stomach and never in combination with any protein food such as milk or meat. Taking amino acids with a carbohydrate source such as fruit juice is recommended by Dr. Harvey M. Ross M.D. who claims that doing this creates an insulin response which helps to facilitate transportation of the substance to brain cells.

This trio of amino acids act as precursors to the synthesis of brain amines. When the body suffers from a lack of any of these amines or neurotransmitters, a drop in mood can occur and depression can result. Research done at MIT has concluded that tyrosine and tryptophan play a profound role in determining the rate at which 4 crucial brain chemicals are produced. These amino acids, directly effect blood levels of these mood controlling neurotransmitters, especially serotonin.

Amino acid therapy works by creating an excess of amino acids which, in turn, forces the body to create increased amounts of neurotransmitters like serotonin. As a result, feelings of depression or melancholy are directly impacted. Technically, drugs like Prozac are designed to accomplish the same goal, which is to elevate these brain chemicals, thereby creating a feeling of well being.

In an issue of *Psychology Today* published in December of 1974, Brian Weiss reported that tyrosine and tryptophan have to compete with other amino acids in order to be transported from the blood to the brain. As a result, under certain circumstances, such as poor diets, serotonin may not get to brain cells.[38] The implications of these findings is that long-term malnutrition has a direct effect on the production of mood altering brain chemicals, like serotonin. L-tryptophan showed great promise in treating not only depression but eating disorders, insomnia, and anxiety as well.

TRYPTOPHAN

Tryptophan is also particularly useful in treating depression in people who experience carbohydrate cravings. As discussed previously, low serotonin levels in the brain may result in these cravings. As a result, if tryptophan is available, eating meals that are carbohydrate rich and low in protein helps to raise serotonin levels even more. If you take tryptophan and eat this way, most of the other amino acids that compete with tryptophan for transport into brain cells will be reduced, therefore enabling tryptophan to increase. As a result, serotonin levels will rise as well. Consuming whole grains such as brown rice, corn, buckwheat, whole wheat and oatmeal and certain vegetables will increase blood and brain levels of tryptophan.

In a study of the connection between tryptophan and depression, the amino acid was administered to 11 patients so severely depressed that they required hospitalization. After a month, 7 of the 11 had significantly less guilt, anxiety, insomnia and weight loss. The overall depressive states of the 11 as determined by standard psychiatric tests dropped by 38 %.[39] Interestingly, those that had the highest blood tryptophan levels, had improved the most.

Barbara Reed, Ph.D., in the book *Food, Teens and Behavior* states: "The body manufactures serotonin from the amino acid tryptophan...a nutrient present in meat and other protein foods...Serotonin deficiencies can be caused by a diet that is poor in tryptophan." One theory proposes that the prevalence of corn, which is tryptophan deficient, in the American diet may account for decreases in serotonin. The American consumption of corn has skyrocketed over the last 50 years. It is not uncommon to consume corn flakes, corn oil, corn oil margerines, corn starch, and corn meal in the form of chips etc. in one day. Corn, in many scenarios has replaced whole wheat, which was a good natural source of tryptophan.

While meat also provides tryptophan, it contains a wide range of other amino acids which compete with eachother. Consequently, a diet which is high in meat does not ensure increased levels of tryptophan in the brain.

Priscilla Slagel, M.D. who wrote a book on the treatment of depression with amino acids and vitamins in 1987 points out that taking amino acids other than tryptophan in therapeutic doses can also act as effective treatments for depression. Her book goes into specific detail on the treatment of depression through amino acid therapy. Her approach utilizes tryptophan, tyrosine, vitamin B-complex, vitamin C and a good multivitamin and mineral supplement. She also discusses the advantages of adding L-phenylalanine or D, L-phenylalanine during the course of treatment. For the current status of tryptophan, see the end of this section.

TYROSINE

Tyrosine, like tryptophan plays a significant role in boosting brain neurotransmitters directly responsible for mood. L-tyrosine can help to alleviate stress by increasing the body's production of adrenaline, which causes a rise in dopamine levels. If a lack of tyrosine exists, insufficient levels of norepinephrine can result. Consequently, a deficiency of this neurotransmitter can cause mood dips and downcast feelings.

Several doctors and psychiatrists have referred to tyrosine as a valuable treatment for ordinary depression and for the mood swings associated with PMS. Dr. Oscar Janiger, M.D. his book a *Different Kind of Healing* comments:

"I've had great results with tyrosine. It's like a natural antidepressant and is a precursor to the neurotransmitter norepinephrine. Once the right dosage is determined, it usually works really well for people with mild depression or severe mood swings especially if you add B-vitamins."[40]

The American Journal of Psychiatry relates another case in which a thirty-year old woman who had suffered for several years from depression and had actually become worse with drug therapy finally tried tyrosine. A team of doctors from Boston and Cambridge gave her tyrosine supplements. The journal reports that after only two weeks, her condition improved dramatically"...she felt better than she had in years and showed striking improvement in mood, self-esteem, sleep, energy level, anxiety and somatic (physical) complaints"[41]

Cases such as this one may be challenged by some doctors who would assume her improvement was a result of the placebo effect. This same woman was given a placebo which was substituted for tyrosine without her knowledge. After one week, her depression began to return. After 18 days, she was more severely depressed than she had been prior to taking the tyrosine.

If you decide to try tyrosine, avoid eating meals that are rich in carbohydrates, which will tend to reduce its effectiveness. Eating meals that are higher in protein when taking tyrosine is recommended, an approach that is the opposite of the suggested diet that boosts tryptophan function. Obviously, the choice to take either tryptophan or tyrosine depends on your particular type of depression. You have to determine if you are a carbohydrate craver or not. You may have to experiment with both treatments to find the best method for you.

PHENYLALANINE

Phenylalanine is also considered an effective antidepressant in that like tyrosine and tryptophan, it acts as precursor to the amines that comprise neurotransmitters in the brain. According to Jose A. Yaryura-Tobias, M.D., phenylalanine converts to phenylethylamine in the body, which is a natural antidepressant.[42] L-phenylalanine can actually convert to tyrosine and it also contributes to the formation of 2-PEA which is believed to be a neurotransmitter which is closely tied with norepinephrine. Some studies show that depressed people lack 2-PEA. Tyrosine is commonly used over phenylalanine because it is better tolerated by most people. If you try phenylalanine, you may feel agitated and nervous. Allergic reactions to phenylalanine are more common than to other amino acids. In some cases, combing tyrosine and phenylalanine may be desireable. If you are concerned about the possible side-effects of using amino acids consider the following. In her experience with using amino acids for depression, Dr. Slagle has stated that, "...in all the years I have been treating depression with amino acids, I have never had to discontinue the treatment because of side-effects. I have, at most, had to modify the tyrosine and phenylalanine usage in cases of pre-existing high blood pressure."[43]

THE CHOCOLATE CONNECTION

Interestingly, the phenylalanine link to depression may help to explain why some women experience intense cravings for chocolate. Anecdotal studies have suggested that frequently, women who suffer from depression consistently crave chocolate. Chocolate contains high concentrations of PEA or phenylalanine which has amphetamine-like stimulant properties which are considered antidepressive substances. When you feel like you could almost kill for something chocolate, your body may be trying to tell you something.

The traditional association between chocolates and romance may be based on the feelings of well being the phenylalanine creates. Low blood levels of phenylalanine and tyrosine have both been found in depressed patients. Anyone who suffers from PMS will probably tell you that their craving for chocolate almost becomes pathological. If you find yourself ransacking your house for an old, stale chocolate or mixing up cocoa and sugar as a mid-afternoon snack, you may be low in phenylalanine. More importantly, if you are low in phenylalanine or tyrosine, you may be susceptible to depression.

HOW TO USE AMINO ACIDS

In order for amino acid therapy to work as a treatment for depression, certain amounts must be taken. Because long term side-effects of taking amino acids have not be researched over long periods of time, caution must be used. Current information suggests that amino acids are far safer than antidepressant drugs. Most doctors who use amino acids for depression will determine exact dosages on an individual basis.

In any event, amino acids should not be given to young children, elderly people or anyone taking MAO antidepressant drugs without professional consultation and guidance. If you are taking MAO inhibitor drugs, taking tyrosine can raise your blood pressure. It is also recommended that if you want to try taking amino acids, you may have to find a doctor who is willing to work with you. Keep in mind that amino acid therapy needs to be carefully monitored. Supplementing amino acids with vitamin B-6 is also recommended.

Vitamin B-6 boosts the body's amino acids and may allow for smaller of amounts of tryptophan and tyrosine to be used. A vitamin B-6 deficiency causes a large amount of available tryptophan to be converted to by-products, which may actually cause the level of serotonin to decline.[44] When you begin taking amino acids, you may feel worse at first. Be assured, that this is a common reaction. Patrician Slagle, M.D. has found that the combination of amino acids and vitamin therapy is usually effective within the first two weeks of use. She points out that most antidepressant medication takes four to six weeks to take effect.

To be most effective, amino acids should be taken at the proper time each day. Taking amino acids on a empty stomach is recommended and they should not be taken with any protein food such as milk etc. Taking amino acids with a small amount of fruit juice to enhance its transportation is also suggested.

You don't have to be a rocket scientist to realize that the body's balance and utilization of neurotransmitters depends on the delicate and complex interaction of foods, amino acids, vitamins and minerals. Tryptophan, tyrosine and phenylalanine are the amino acids that function as precursors to the brain chemicals directly responsible for determining our mood status. If we do not get adequate amount of these precursors through our diets, depression can occur. It's that simple.

If you decide to use amino acid supplements, don't expect an overnight cure. Your symptoms may not abate for several weeks, however the benefits of natural treatments like amino acids are well worth the wait. It must be stressed that when you use natural therapies, results sometimes take longer that with prescription drugs. Remember that while drugs can have quick and dramatic effects, they can also come with significant risks.

At the same time, all amino acids should also be used judiciously. There may be some risk of elevating blood pressure, if you use phenylalanine. Ideally, any amino acid therapy program should be employed under a doctor's supervision.

The encouraging news is that amino acid therapy may provide safe and natural relief from depression, its readily available and relatively inexpensive. For more information on amino acid therapy, doses etc. for depression see:

The Way Up From Down, Priscilla Slagle, M.D. Random House, 1987.

NOTE: TRYPTOPHAN: IT'S CURRENT STATUS

Using amino acids as a natural alternative treatment for depression was recently dealt a blow when L-tryptophan was removed from the market after some serious side-effects resulted from a particular batch of the amino acid. Further investigation concluded that a production flaw was responsible for the tainted tryptophan. Unfortunately, even with this evidence, the FDA has not permitted the sales of L-tryptophan to the general public.

For over three decades, tryptophan was safely used by millions of people for conditions such as insomnia and depression. In 1988, a very rare condition called Eosinophilia-Myalgia Syndrome (EMS) was traced to a contaminated batch of tryptophan. As a result, on November 17, 1989, The FDA ordered that all tryptophan should be pulled from the market.

All cases of EMS were subsequently traced to Showa Denko, a Japanese petrochemical company that supplied over 50 percent of tryptophan used in the United States. In 1988, Denko altered its filtration processes which resulted in the contaminated tryptophan. Despite the fact that the source of the contamination was discovered, all tryptophan was removed. The fact that it had been used safely for over 30 years was not significant to the FDA. Numerous studies proving that the cases of EMS in question were caused by the temporary contamination of this particular source of tryptophan did not settle the issue. According to an August, 1990 article in the *New England Journal of Medicine,* researchers at the Center of Disease Control concluded: "Our data indicate that the 1989 outbreak of the syndrome was caused by the consumption of tryptophan that was manufactured by a single company."[45]

The FDA ban on tryptophan continues today. In addition, the FDA is considering making all amino acids prescription medications or removing them all together from the market place. If amino acids were only available through a doctor's prescription, you can imagine what would happen to their price. What's even more troubling is that amino acids are considered nutrients. Placing these nutrients out of the reach of the public into pharmaceutical distributorship puts all nutrients at risk.

Patrician Slagle M.D. puts it this way:" If tryptophan is dangerous, then why not ban milk, turkey, and other foods with naturally high amounts of tryptophan? Tryptophan helps the body to make more serotonin. Normal metabolic processes regulate serotonin production and prevent the body from making too much, Contrast this to the powerful new and controversial drugs approved and defended by the FDA, such as Prozac, which increases the brain's serotonin levels and can override the natural metabolic process which would stop the over accumulation of serotonin. Such drugs can sometimes cause an abnormal excess of serotonin and may have significant debilitating side-effects." [46]

Her point is well taken. Unfortunately, the health food industry is subject to this kind of discrimination. You can be sure that if a batch of Coca Cola was contaminated, all Coke would not be indefinitely banned throughout the country. Tryptophan has not been allowed to return to store shelves regardless of the fact that the issue of its contamination has been put to rest. The irony of it all is that an effective treatment against EMS, the contaminant in question, is tryptophan itself. [47]

The message of the tryptophan controversy is clear. Let's all defend our right to purchase and use natural health care products. Elected government officials and agencies need to know that freedom of choice applies to treating disease also.

DEPRESSION, VITAMINS
AND MINERALS

*"Your foods shall be your remedies, and your
remedies shall be your foods"*

Hippocrates

In a 1960's a Psychiatrist found that adding megavitamin therapy
to the standard medical treatment of three schizophrenic patients had
some striking results. Each was placed on a low blood sugar diet
supplemented with megadoses of niacin or niacinamide, in
combination with Vitamin C, B-6 and E. One patient in particular
improved so dramatically that her life took a swift upturn and
electric shock treatments were no longer necessary. This psychiatrist
eventually developed a private practice which uses nutritional
therapy consisting of vitamins and diet to treat patients who would
otherwise be taking mood altering drugs.

For decades, experts in the health and nutrition field have been
passionately emphasizing that what we eat clearly affects our
physical health, not to mention our mental outlook. As mentioned
previously, our nation may be the most overfed and under nourished
country on earth. Nutrient deficiencies can abound, even here in the
land of plenty, and those deficiencies can make us feel perpetually
sad.

More and more psychiatrists are looking at the psychological
effects of nutrient depletion, however, their numbers are too few.
Regardless of the fact that the medical profession is notorious for
dragging its feet about such things, the use of vitamins and minerals
to treat illness cannot be ignored.

Sadly enough, doctors who are willing to use vitamin therapy
are few. Chances are, if your ask your physician if he thinks vitamin
therapy might help your depression, he'll really think you've gone
off the deep end. While the information in this book never proposes
that all mental disorders are the result of nutritional deficiencies, in
many cases, vitamins play a profound role in facilitating a cure.

Again, if you feel your diet is adequately supplying you with all the nutrients you need to be healthy, consider the following: Some psychologically disturbed individuals suffer from the abnormal metabolism of one or more vitamins, minerals, amino acids or fatty acids which can increase their particular nutrient requirements far above the minimal standards set in the RDA. In other words, you may think your diet is satisfactory, when, in fact, you may be malnourished.

VITAMINS: DO WE GET WHAT WE REALLY NEED FOR OPTIMAL HEALTH

Many of us may be suffering from borderline B-vitamin deficiencies that we have no way of knowing exist. If you go to your doctor and complain of unexplained depression or fatigue, nutrient deficiencies are rarely suspected. Even if they were, testing would more than likely reveal nothing. Many experts including some doctors are of the opinion that these types of subtle deficiencies are much more common than anyone imagined. Teenagers who eat junk food and senior citizens, who often try to save money by cutting their food budget are especially susceptible to this type of B-vitamin deficiency.

Many health care professionals believe that the American diet is deficient in several nutrients which are considered low as set by the RDA. In addition, if you smoke or drink or are exposed to a variety of environmental toxins, the vitamins you do get may be impaired or even destroyed. Robert Picker M.D. a California physician says: "Some people have been brainwashed by traditional medicine into believing that we are getting all the nutrients we need in our average diet, but there are numerous large-scale studies to counter that fallacy. They show there is a large percentage of the American public that is below the Recommended Dietary Allowance (RDA) for many key nutrients, including some of the B-vitamins."

Deficiencies of vitamins B-1, B-6, C, and A, along with folic acid, niacin, magnesium, copper and iron can all cause depression by influencing the synthesis of serotonin and norepinephrine. Virtually any nutrient deficiency can result in depression. The following table lists the behavioral effects of 8 nutrient deficiencies:

DEFICIENT VITAMIN	RESULTING BEHAVIOR
ASCORBIC ACID (VITAMIN C)	DEPRESSION, HYSTERIA, HYPOCHONDRIASIS, LASSITUDE. CONFUSION
BIOTIN	DEPRESSION, EXTREME LASSITUDE, SOMNOLENCE
CYANOCOBALAMIN (VITAMIN B-12)	DEPRESSION, PSYCHOTIC STATES, IRRITABILITY, CONFUSION, MEMORY LOSS, HALLUCINATIONS, DELUSIONS, PARANOIA, MOOD SWINGS
FOLIC ACID	DEPRESSION, APATHY, INSOMNIA, IRRITABILITY, DELIRIUM, FORGETFULNESS, PSYCHOSIS, DEMENTIA
NIACIN (VITAMIN B-3)	DEPRESSION, MANIA, MEMORY DEFICITS, APATHY, ANXIETY, HYPERIRRITABILITY, EMOTIONAL INSTABILITY, POOR CONCENTRATION
PANTOTHENIC ACID (VITAMIN B-5)	DEPRESSION, RESTLESSNESS, IRRITABILITY, FATIGUE, QUARRELSOMENESS
PYRIDOXINE (VITAMIN B-6)	DEPRESSION, IRRITABILITY, NERVOUSNESS, INSOMNIA, POOR DREAM RECALL
THIAMINE (VITAMIN B-1)	DEPRESSION, APATHY, ANXIETY, IRRITABILITY, MEMORY LOSS, PERSONALITYCHANGES, EMOTIONAL INSTABILITY
RIBOFLAVIN (VITAMIN B-2)	DEPRESSION, INSOMNIA, MENTAL SLUGGISHNESS

RDA STANDARDS MAY NOT BE REALISTIC

The nutritional treatment of depression assumes that what we may think are adequate levels of vitamins and minerals, may in fact be too low for our particular systemic needs. This does not imply that megadoses of vitamins are always a good thing. What it suggests is that what we have considered acceptable dietary habits, may not be supplying us nutrient levels needed for optimal health, not just for survival.

For example, in order to receive the maximum nutritional benefit from foods that we consume our diet would typically have to consist of several portions of whole grain products, several servings of fresh, raw fruits and vegetables, legumes, nuts, or other protein sources and adequate, absorbable sources of calcium. Who eats like this every day? Do you?

Several studies that analyze diet have discovered that it's common to find at least three to four nutrient deficiencies even by RDA standards and significantly more by ideal setpoint charts. Ideally, we should get what we need from our diet. In reality, this is rarely the case. Nutrient insufficiencies abound, with the B-vitamins being particularly vulnerable. Question: What is one of the most prevalent symptoms of a B-vitamin deficiency? Depression.

THE B VITAMINS AND DEPRESSION

VITAMIN B-6

One study of fifteen pregnant women who were depressed revealed that they all suffered from some degree of vitamin B-6 deficiency.[48] Interestingly, several other studies have found that frequently, women who take birth control pills and become depressed have low levels of B-6.[49] In light of these studies, the *British Journal of Psychiatry* concluded that "more attention should be paid to assessing the...pyridoxine (vitamin B-6) status of the mentally ill in the hope of detecting and correcting deficiencies."

There can be no question that vitamin B-6 levels strongly correlate with mood disorders. Research supports the fact that as many as 20 percent of people hospitalized for depression are lacking vitamin B-6. What is fascinating is that they showed no physical signs of this deficiency.[50] While vitamin B-6 is readily available in most foods, deficiencies can result from taking certain drugs including, oral contraceptives, exposure to a variety of pollutants, and ingesting too much sugar or caffeine. Ironically, MAO inhibitors, which are antidepressant medications also deplete vitamin B-6 reserves.

Scientific evidence that B-6 can effectively treat depression came from an English study done by P.W. Adams, M.D. and his staff. They carefully observed 22 depressed women who were all taking birth control pills. Because birth control pills can deplete the body of vitamin B-6, Dr. Adams assumed that a deficiency was related to the onset of depression. Half of these women were found to be vitamin B-6 deficient, and when given supplements experienced relief from their depression.[51]

Several other studies done at the Virginia Polytechnic Institute and State University and at the National Institute of Mental Health have confirmed that plasma levels of vitamin B-6 were approximately 48% lower in depressed patients. While some doctors refute the validity of the vitamin B-6 connection to severe depression, the statistics cannot be ignored or misinterpreted. Clearly, scientific evidence points to the fact that a vitamin B-6 deficiency may be quite commonplace in some depressed individuals.

Women who suffer from post-partum depression have a higher risk for developing a vitamin B deficiency. Some women become deficient in Vitamin B-6 during the course of their pregnancy. Consequently, after the baby is born they experience an intense period of melancholia. In some cases, where a lack of vitamin B-6 was not a factor, deficiencies in vitamin B-12 or folate were discovered. At any rate, keeping the body supplied with adequate amounts of the B vitamins cannot be over-emphasized in helping to prevent or treat certain cases of unexplained depression.

It is also vital that we all remember that blood and urine tests don't always conclusively represent what may be going on in brain biochemistry. It has been pointed out that a vitamin B-6 deficiency could conceivably exist in the brain, even when blood or urine levels present as normal.[52] Again, the reliability of certain lab tests is dubious.

People who have abnormal enzymes in the brain that would

require unusually high amounts of vitamin B-6 to function may develop depression even if they have adequate supplies of vitamin B-6 in the brain. Even in these cases, certain doctors believe that supplementation of B-6 would still be helpful. Without question, the B-vitamins play an enormous role in determining mental outlook and health.

VITAMIN B12

Vitamin B-12 can also be used in your antidepression nutrient program. A very small amount of vitamin B-12 is absorbed by the body either through food or nutrient supplementation. Consequently, taking an oral supplement of B-12 is not recommended. Dr. Slagle uses sublingual vitamin B-12 which are tablets designed to melt under your tongue. She recommends using this form of B-12 first thing in the morning to prevent the onset of a "low" period.

It's easy enough to supplement one's diet with B-vitamins which have no harmful side-effects and are relatively inexpensive. Women who take the pill should be advised by their physicians that taking B vitamins can help eliminate the depression that sometimes occurs as a side-effect. The message is clear...get yourself a good supply of B vitamins and take them for the rest of your life.

FOLIC ACID

Folic acid is another essential nutrient for treating depression. It works synergistically with vitamin B-12 and contributes to neurotransmitter production in the brain. A deficiency of folic acid can also cause you to feel depressed. Folate is a member of the vitamin B family and is absolutely essential for the proper functioning of the central nervous system. Research done at the Royal Victoria Hospital in Montreal clearly supports the fact that if you become deficient in folic acid and get depressed, taking supplements can make you feel 100% better.[53]

Green leafy vegetables are the main source of folic acid, however high cooking temperatures destroy over half the available vitamin content. Due to its vulnerability to heat, folic acid deficiencies are the most common kind. Some physicians actually assess your overall nutritional status by checking your folate level.

That's how vital it is.

If you think you're getting enough folic acid, think again. Poor eating, which includes many weight reducing diets can be responsible for low folate levels. In addition, taking aspirin, barbiturates, anticonvulsants, oral contraceptives and other drugs can inhibit the absorption of folic acid into the body. Early signs of a folic acid deficiency are fatigue, and lethargy. Later depression, burning feet, and restless legs can occur.

Blood levels of folate are frequently low in a significant number of depressed individuals. A folic acid deficiency is the most common nutritional deficiency in the world. As many as 30 percent of psychiatric patients are low in folate. In one study, 67 percent of elderly patients admitted to a psychiatric facility were deficient in folic acid.[54] Again, the relationship of malnutrition and geriatric depression should not be minimized. Unfortunately, it is rarely addressed.

VITAMIN B3

Niacin (Vitamin B-3) is also necessary for the proper metabolism of tryptophan and should also be supplemented. Along with niacin and vitamin B-6, vitamin B-1 (thiamine) is also essential to activate the energy transport system of the body.

Interestingly, with all this emphasis on B-vitamins and mental health, remember that a vitamin B deficiency not only causes depression but can itself be a side-effect of it. Depressed people eat poorly. What else is new? Consequently, malnutrition can easily develope. Which came first then, the depression or the deficiency? To make matters worse, penicillamine, cigarette smoke, and a whole host of pollutants and toxic chemicals can destroy vitamin B stores in the body. Is it farfetched to assume that the pervasive and widespread contamination of our environments with vitamin B antagonists may be responsible, in part, for the ever-escalating incidence of depression? Regardless of the answer, the value of the B-complex vitamins in the prevention and treatment of depression should be carefully considered.

Just to bring this point home, consider some of the substances and environmental conditions that destroy B-vitamins and various minerals: caffeine, tobacco, alcohol, stress, fever, heat, sugar, food processing, ultraviolet light, antibiotics, anticonvulsants, radiation, estrogen, birth control pills, cortisone, aspirin, diuretics, antacids, some laxatives, some sleeping pills, barbiturates, cooking heat, high protein diets, mineral oil, chorine, rancid fats and oils, oxalic acid, heavy metals, aluminum, chlorine etc. etc. etc.

If you decide to take vitamin B supplements for depression, be advised that when you first start, you may experience an initial period where you feel even worse. For reasons that remain unclear, sometimes an initial rise in B-6 levels can cause your depression to intensify. In these cases, experimenting with reduced dosages will be necessary. Remember that creating a working equilibrium between all vitamins and minerals is the ultimate goal.

There are several theories suggesting that brain amines may become more imbalanced as the body adjusts to a rise in certain vitamins, and that enzyme malfunctions may react negatively to the presence of the vitamin. These reasons are purely speculative, however, anyone who decides to take vitamin B-6, should do so under a doctor's supervision. For those people who do feel worse, taking niacinamide and tryptophan may improve symptoms.[55]

In our discussion of the value of vitamins in maintaining mental health, it is interesting to note that one report in medical journals links high levels of a mineral called vanadium to depression. Taking vitamin C helps to detoxify vanadium. It seems reasonable to assume that there may be other toxic substances that we inadvertently ingest or breathe that may also cause mood disorders. In any event, taking vitamin C is a wise practice regardless of whether you're depressed or not. It seems that this vitamin is full of surprises and continues to impress scientists with its long list of benefits.

VITAMIN C AND BIOFLAVONOIDS

Vitamin C with bioflavonoids is required to synthesize norepinephrine and serotonin. Bioflavonoids in combination with vitamin C provide the body with a very impressive defense system against oxidation or the breakdown of norepinephrine in brain cells. New studies also suggest that bioflavonoids promote better memory and reduce insomnia.

Bioflavonoids are nutrients that cannot be produced by the

human body, therefore, they have to be obtained from foods or supplements. While RDA requirements for bioflavonoids are usually met by a decent diet, the therapeutic use of bioflavonoids holds tremendous promise for a variety of ailments including neurological disorders.

Bioflavonoids have the ability to pass through the blood-brain barrier, thereby serving as antioxidants to brain cells. Several scientific studies strongly suggest that antioxidants can help restore normal neurochemical balance in the brain following surgery or trauma.[56] Oxidative stress is repeatedly cited and implicated in a wide variety of nervous system disorders.

Bioflavonoids are chemical constituents of pulp and the rind of citrus fruits, green peppers, apricots, cherries, grapes, papayas, tomatoes, and broccoli. Bioflavonoids are not really considered vitamins, however, their value is enormous. For one thing, they increase the body's ability to absorb vitamin C to a great extent. It's important to always take vitamin C together with bioflavonoids as they greatly enhance each other.

Minerals are also intrinsically involved in the preservation of wellness. Many experts believe that calcium and magnesium have the power to help chase away melancholia in some individuals. It is interesting to learn that depressed people who took lithium and improved also showed a rise in their magnesium levels, while the magnesium levels of those who tried lithium and stayed depressed stayed the same.[57]

CALCIUM/MAGNESIUM

The body is extremely sensitive to fluctuations in calcium levels. Brain cells cannot function normally if there is an excess or a lack of calcium. Dr. August F. Daro, an obstetrician and gynecologist in Chicago gives his depressed patients calcium and magnesium as a standard treatment. He states that "many depressed men and women are short on calcium and magnesium...I put them on a combination of 400 milligrams of calcium and 200 milligrams of magnesium a day. These minerals sedate the nervous system, and most of the depressed patients feel much better while taking them. Calcium and magnesium especially take care of premenstrual depression."[58] The question then, is: are you getting enough calcium and magnesium?

In the February 20th 1985 issue of *Biological Psychiatry* a study of forty-one unmedicated psychiatric patients indicated that eleven women who had attempted suicide had significantly lower cerebrospinal fluid levels of magnesium than those who had not attempted suicide. As a result, conclusions that magnesium may be required to maintain normal serotonin activity in the brain have been drawn.[60]

Comparable studies of other psychiatric patients who experienced depression, schizophrenia and sleep disturbances also pointed to low magnesium blood levels. Like phenylalanine, a lack of magnesium can create a chocolate craving. Taking magnesium supplements for PMS symptoms has been recommended to help stem the mood swings that are typical for some women. The implications here are worth investigating. Obviously, changes in estrogen levels may affect magnesium levels which may affect mood.

There is also considerable speculation that too much of one mineral and not enough of another can create depressed mental states. Some medical doctors who believe that the most common mineral imbalance among people who are depressed was an excess of copper and a lack of zinc and manganese. In these cases, zinc and manganese are administered in combination with vitamin B-6 to initiate the excretion of copper in the urine. Using chealated zinc is recommended.

ENVIRONMENTAL DRAINS ON
VITAMIN AND MINERAL STORES

Due to the nature of our environments and our poor dietary habits, it is very easy to become nutrient deficient. If you believe you are getting adequate amounts of vitamins and minerals from your diet, you may be deluding yourself. Any of the following situations can cause vitamin and mineral depletion:

- pregnancy or nursing
- stress
- consuming caffeine
- using tobacco
- several drugs including: birth control pills, aspirin, tranquilizers, and sleeping pills
- dieting
- exposure to pesticides
- air pollution
- drinking fluoridated or chlorinated water
- adolescence
- physical illness
- surgery or any kind of trauma, emotional or physical
- gastrointestinal disorders
- illicit drugs
- excess consumption of junk foods including white sugar and white flour

How many of us are protected from these nutrient robbers?

SUMMARY OF SPECIFIC VITAMINS AND MINERALS USED IN TREATING DEPRESSION

VITAMIN B-6 (pyridoxine)

Of all the B vitamins, vitamin B-6 has the most profound affect on the regulation of moods. Its correlation with depression cannot be ignored. If you suffer from depression, you may be deficient in B6, a condition which is common to people who suffer from a variety of mental disorders.

Vitamin B-6 enables proper amino acid utilization which is vital for the healthy maintenance of brain chemicals. Vitamin B-6 participates in the regulation and absorption of amino acids in the digestive system and also contributes to the breakdown of carbohydrates and fats. Without adequate supplies of vitamin B-6. the enzyme systems of the body could not function properly.

Vitamin B-6 is also effective for PMS. Various scientific studies suggest that using daily doses of vitamin B-6 of between 200 and 800 mg. per day can significantly curb PMS symptoms.

If you want to use vitamin B-6 for depression, obtain the active coenzyme form for optimal effectiveness. Take vitamin B-6 along with other B vitamins and keep them all at approximately the same dosage to ensure they will complement each other properly.

FOOD SOURCES: BREWER'S YEAST, BLACKSTRAP MOLASSES, LIVER, HERRING, SALMON, NUTS, BROWN RICE, SOYBEANS, EGGS, BANANAS, AVOCADOS, GRAPES AND PEARS.

VITAMIN B-1 (thiamine)

The most classic symptoms of depression: fatigue, insomnia, irritability are all markers of a deficiency of vitamin B-1. B-1 is required for the brain to utilize carbohydrates, which is its primary source of fuel. Vitamin B-1, like B-6 also participates in the production of certain neurotransmitters, and helps to increase our stamina by supplying our body with energy. Make sure to take this vitamin in combination with other B vitamins.

FOOD SOURCES: WHEAT GERM, WHEAT BRAN, BREWER'S YEAST, BLACKSTRAP MOLASSES, SOYBEANS, PORK, LIVER, NUTS, OATMEAL, AND POULTRY

VITAMIN B-3 (niacin)

Anxiety, mental slowing and depression are just a few symptoms of a vitamin B-3 deficiency. There has been some speculation that if the diet is deficient in niacin, tryptophan stores may be used to synthesize it thereby creating a deficit for serotonin production in the brain. Like B-1, this vitamin works to help facilitate proper brain function and metabolism. It participates in breaking down nutrients for our body's use and is also involved in the synthesis of certain hormones.

Vitamin B-3 can have a calming effect on the brain. Apparently, it binds to some of the same locations in brain cells that prescription tranquilizers do. Take normal amount of this vitamin for depression as part of the vitamin B complex group.

SOURCES: PEANUTS, RACE BRAN, ORGAN MEATS, TUNA, HALIBUT, SWORDFISH, BREWER'S YEAST, AVOCADOS, ASPARAGUS, BEANS, POTATOES, NUTS, WHOLE GRAINS AND MUSHROOMS

VITAMIN B-5 (pantothenic acid)

This vitamin is essential for good mental health in that it promotes the uptake of amino acids so crucial to proper brain function and participates in hormone production as well. It plays a part in the formation of acetylcholine, a neurotransmitter which if depleted, can also initiate depression

SOURCES: BREWER'S YEAST, BLACKSTRAP MOLASSES, HERRING, SALMON, LIVER, BROWN RICE, SOYBEANS, BANANAS, AVOCADOS, PEARS AND GRAPES

VITAMIN B-12 (cyanocobalamin or hydroxocobalamin)

Adequate supplies of vitamin B-12 are necessary in order to maintain a healthy nervous system. This vitamin works to keep neurons working properly, which explains why it is so crucial to the maintenance of good mental health.

Vitamin B-12 seems especially effective against the type of depression and fatigue that can occur after an infection or other form of stress on the body.

Because the vitamin is often poorly absorbed, some doctors have recommended using a sublingual form rather than a pill. Vitamin B-12 injections are also available. The side-effects of a vitamin B-12 deficiency are significant to say the least. Severe depression in combination with mental fatigue, difficulty concentrating and hallucinations can occur.

SOURCES: ORGAN MEATS, EGG YOLKS, CLAMS, SALMON, CRAB, SARDINES, OYSTERS, HERRING

FOLIC ACID

A number of recent studies have shown that psychiatric patients have lower folic acid levels that normal subjects, and that a minimum of 20 percent of depressed inpatients with no anemia have unusually low levels.[61] Folic acid is essential for the proper formation of serotonin and norepinephrine in the brain. Because folic acid facilitates adrenal gland secretion, it is also necessary to help the body cope with stress.

Some studies have shown that elderly people are notoriously low in folic acid which may help to explain why depression and other mental disorders are so rampant among older segments of the population.

If you become deficient in folic acid, you will feel depressed, tired and mentally dull. Remember that alcohol interferes with folic acid, as well as anticonvulsant drugs and birth control pills. Folic acid also help to boost estrogen levels, which may be desireable for menopausal women. A folic acid deficiency during pregnancy can increase the likelihood of premature delivery and birth defects.

SOURCES: LIVER, BREWER'S YEAST, SPINACH, ASPARAGUS, LENTILS, LIMA BEANS, NAVY BEANS, GREEN VEGETABLES, ALMONDS, PEANUTS, FILBERTS, WALNUTS, OATS, WHEAT AND RYE

VITAMIN C with Bioflavonoids

Vitamin C may well be called the wonder vitamin. It participates in so many health promoting functions of the body. Regarding mental health, vitamin C is involved in the action of the amino acids, phenylalanine and tyrosine, two essential precursors to the formation of the neurotransmitters needed to prevent depression.

Vitamin C can also stimulate the adrenal glands. Perhaps one of its most important functions regarding depression, is its role as a detoxifier. So many of the chemicals and pollutants we are routinely exposed to may be unseen causes of mood swings. Vitamin C helps to neutralize these harmful substances.

Bioflavonoids are considered powerful antioxidants that can promote healing within brain tissue and help to restore normal levels of neurochemicals. Together with vitamin C, bioflavonoids provide invaluable support to the maintenance of brain cell integrity.

Vitamin C is easily destroyed through processing, heat, exposure to pollutants, toxic metals, chemicals, tobacco and various drugs. Keep in mind, however, that the more we are exposed to these environmental hazards, the more vitamin C we require. Oral contraceptives, tetracycline stress, aspirin, pregnancy, nursing, aging, infection, surgery and any injury all increase the body's need for vitamin C.

SOURCES: BROCCOLI, COLLARDS, BRUSSEL SPROUTS, KALE, PARSLEY, GREEN PEPPERS, TURNIP GREENS, BLACK CURRANTS, GUAVA, CITRUS FRUITS, CABBAGE. TOMATOES, CAULIFLOWER AND SPINACH

BIOTIN

Biotin is required for the proper synthesis of serotonin in the brain. Studies have shown that a biotin deficient diet can produce depression, hallucinations and even panic. Fortunately, biotin deficiencies are not common. Keep in mind, however, that if you take high doses of antibiotics, you can develope a biotin deficiency.

SOURCES: BREWER'S YEAST, LOVER, BROWN RICE. WHEAT, CORN, CHICKPEAS, LEGUMES, MUSHROOMS, BARLEY, NUTS, SARDINES, SALMON AND MACKEREL

MAGNESIUM

This mineral is another coenzyme that is required for the proper formation of brain amines or neurotransmitters. In order for the B vitamins to be effectively assimilated, sufficient levels of magnesium must be present. A whole host of psychological symptoms can result from a lack of magnesium and particularly low levels have been discovered in suicidal patients. Most American diets are low in magnesium. In addition, smoking, drinking, physical and mental stress, eating a diet high in fat, protein, salt and phosphates or drinking soft water can also decrease magnesium stores.

SOURCES: WHEAT GERM AND BRAN, RAW ALMONDS, CASHEWS, BLACKSTRAP MOLASSES, BREWER'S YEAST, SOYBEANS, SESAME SEED, WILD RICE, OATS, RYE, MILLET, BARLEY, PEAS, CARROTS AND BEET GREENS

MANGANESE

This mineral is needed for the proper formation of neurotransmitters in the brain and also affects pituitary gland function which regulates hormone levels. A lack of manganese can aggravate low blood sugar which in and of itself can predispose one to depression. If you eat a lot of dairy foods, you may be inhibiting manganese assimilation. Ingesting a lot of soft drinks and excess phosphorus which is commonly found in most junk foods can also decrease manganese absorption.

SOURCES: COCONUT, SUNFLOWER SEEDS, NUTS, BARLEY, RYE, BUCKWHEAT, SPLIT PEAS, WHOLE WHEAT, SPINACH, RAISINS, OLIVES, AVOCADOS, BLUEBERRIES

Clearly, it is safe to assume that most of us are suffering from inadequate nutrition. Furthermore, any of us who are battling depression need to heed that very real connection between nutrients and brain function. Those nutrients that we should pay attention to are: the amino acids tryptophan, tyrosine and phenylalanine (refer to chapter on amino acids), the B-vitamins, B-6 specifically, along with folic acid, and biotin, vitamin C, vitamin E, calcium, magnesium, manganese, zinc, iron copper and pancreatic enzymes.

Realizing that most of us are probably nutrient deficient does not justify recklessly taking vitamin and mineral supplements. Balance is crucial and the ideal scenario would be to find a nutritionally oriented physician who could help you design and monitor a vitamin and mineral treatment plan for your depression.

LIGHT AND DEPRESSION

"Light is the first of painters. There is no object so foul that intense light will not make it beautiful."

Ralph Waldo Emerson

Recently, there has been a great deal of interest in the type of depression that is instigated by a lack of exposure to sunlight. It is sometimes referred to as SAD, or seasonal affective disorder. In areas of the world where the days are extremely short, moods and attitudes seem to be directly impacted by this lack of light. James E. Cathey, Ph.D., secretary of the Society for the Advancement of Scandinavian Study says that Scandinavians have been traditionally stereotyped as "dour personalities." He says that people who live in these types of extreme climate have not found a successful way to cope with darkness and cold and continually yearn for the light and warmth of the sun.[62]

On May 16, 1898, Arctic explorer Frederick A. Cook wrote in his journal: "The winter and the darkness have slowly but steadily settled over us...It is not difficult to read on the faces of my companions their thoughts and their moody dispositions...The curtain of blackness which has fallen over the outer world of icy desolation has also descended upon the inner world of our souls. Around the tables...men are sitting about sad and dejected, lost in dreams of melancholy from which now and them, one arouses with an empty attempt at enthusiasm."[63]

It has been estimated that up to 10% of the population experience the "winter blues." Like any other form of depression, its symptoms can be crippling, affecting job performance, and family relationships. While most of us gripe more during the cold, dark months of winter, some of us become plagued with feelings of overwhelming fatigue. We may overeat to compensate for a feeling of emptiness, and our productivity may drop dramatically.

Over the last ten years, studies have closely investigated the impact that a lack of light has on certain individuals. These studies suggest that sunlight deprivation causes a type of depression for some people. Today, more and more psychiatrists and endocrinologists are recognizing the complex effects that light can exert on the human body. What they have found is a lack of light can cause the nervous system to become depressed. This seasonal depression is somewhat different in its symptoms than classical depression.

Significant differences between people who suffer from SAD and other forms of depression is SAD sufferers tend to eat more, turning to carbohydrates or alcohol for mental stimulation, and they tend to oversleep. While a loss of appetite and insomnia are the general rule in standard cases of depression, opposite behaviors can also occur. The fact that a seasonal change can clear up SAD also distinguishes it from typical depression. For a clinically depressed person, even the arrival of Spring fails to exhilarate.

LIGHT AND BIOCHEMISTRY

New studies have indicated that light has a much greater impact on the biochemistry and bio-rhythms of the body than previously thought. Experiments with light exposure have helped to combat the jet lag we experience when we travel and get our days and nights mixed up. In these cases, Japanese researchers have found that people flying from west to east can decrease jet lag by receiving two hours of early morning bright light for the first three days after their arrival.[64]

Shift workers can also be treated similarly. In addition, light therapy has been used to help regulate menstrual periods in some women. Even some blind people are thought to somehow be light sensitive, enabling them to avoid the insomnia which frequently plagues others who are blind and have no way to tell if it's light or dark. It is also believed that light may boost the functions of the immune system, thereby affording greater protection against disease. Light is believed to effect female ovulation, the ability to absorb calcium, and is used to treat jaundice in newborns.

Accordingly, it is now believed that the number of daylight hours we are exposed to indicates to our physical and mental beings the time of day and year it is. This explains in part why our appetites and sleep patterns vary. Light can stimulate or suppress the secretion of hormones which regulate these cycles.

For example, the pineal gland produces a hormone called melatonin, which can produce a desire to sleep in most animals. As day darkens, the pineal gland begins to respond by producing melatonin, which can make us feel drowsy. In addition, melatonin also raises the level of serotonin in the brain.

If you've ever attended a lecture in a dimly lit classroom, you may have become overwhelmed by a sudden desire to sleep. It is believed that the supply of light, which enters the eye either stimulates or suppresses the release of melatonin. When morning light reaches the pineal gland through the eyes, melatonin production is stopped. For this reason, some scientists believe that removing the eyes of totally blind people for cosmetic purposes is not advisable. Even blind eyes can respond to the presence of light in some individuals.

Because the pineal gland is interrelated with the rest of the endocrine system, its function affects the pituitary gland, which in turn affects the thyroid gland, which affects the adrenal glands, etc. etc. In the past, when cycles of light and darkness relied on nature's patterns, human beings responded accordingly, retiring early and rising at dawn. Today, this is no longer the case. The invention of electricity can transform night into day and winter into summer. Conversely, air conditioning, window treatments and tinted glass can protect us from the natural light and warmth of summer months.

There is significant speculation that the reason we still get sleepy even under bright lights late at night is that indoor lighting is not intense enough to trigger the hormonal responses needed to keep us awake. Research has shown that light that is at least 2,500 lux is required to suppress the production of melatonin.[65] The average electric light bulb is approximately 500 lux. The resulting conclusion is that low intensity, artificial light does not satisfy our bodies' requirement for natural sunlight.

Dr. Richard Wurtman, Ph.D. of MIT points out that artificial lights that are typically used to illuminate interiors provide only around one-tenth of the light which would be found outside under one shade tree on a sunny day.

It would seem then that if daylight hours could be extended, a whole variety of mental and physical reactions would result. Studies have concluded that in several countries even the rate of conception increases when daylight hours are the longest. Exposure to sunlight has been found to impact the timing and quality of sleep, appetite fluctuations, sexual activity, the onset of the menstrual cycle, pain endurance and mood.

SYMPTOMS OF SEASONAL AFFECTIVE DISORDER

What does SAD or winter depression feel like? People who suffer from a seasonal mood disorder feel sad, anxious and irritable. They may feel constantly fatigued, oversleep or fall asleep during the day. In addition, they usually crave sweets and junk food, overeat and may experience headaches.

> *"I just can't get up in the morning. Even with the Christmas season approaching, I couldn't seem to muster the energy or enthusiasm I needed to make the holidays special. I feel so melancholy and tired. All I want to do is get under the covers and sleep. When I'm not sleeping, I want to eat. First I'll eat some cookies, then I'll crave some ice cream, then I'll want something salty like potato chips. I've gained weight and that makes me feel even worse. I don't want anybody to see me. I'm also having trouble concentrating and making even simple choices. I feel like a lazy slob but I can't seem to snap out of it."*

These sentiments are typical of a seasonal mood disorder which is characterized by comfort eating, fatigue and oversleeping. Keep in mind that the type of sleep SAD sufferers experience only serves to make them feel more tired. While other physical components may play a role in this type of mood disorder, light starvation is considered the primary causal factor.

Research done at the National Institute of Mental Health, in Bethesda, Maryland by a team of psychiatrists took 30 people with a history of winter depression and summer elation and used light or phototherapy to treat them. Preliminary findings showed that using a special artificial light which approximates the light spectrum of the sun was valuable. This light reproduces the same effect which the longest day of the year creates, and had some very encouraging results. These people used the lights during the winter months for three hours every morning and every night. For some, the response was dramatic and improvement significant.

Researchers have come away from studies such as this one believing that human beings have seasonal rhythms that are largely determined by the presence of sunlight. People who suffer from SAD, may be unaware that something as simple as morning exposure to bright light may make them feel 100 percent better.

Dr. Thomas Wehr and Dr. Norman Rosenthal, both medical doctors at the National Institute of Mental Health created an artificial "spring" as treatment for a 63-year-old manic-depressive patient. During the first week of December, they woke him up at 6:00 AM and exposed him to extremely bright artificial light for three hours. At 4:00 PM, they repeated the exposure for another three hours. Technically, what they did was artificially lengthen his days. They continued this therapy for ten days. After only four days, this man felt much better and began to come out of his social withdrawal.[66]

NEUROTRANSMITTERS, PMS, FOOD CRAVINGS AND LIGHT

What is particularly interesting considering other topics discussed in this book is that SAD may also be related to hormonal deficiencies in certain people which supports what we already know: that a deficiency in serotonin and dopamine, two critical neurotransmitters in the brain may increase one's susceptibility to depression. During the winter months, generally speaking, serotonin levels in the brain can be at their lowest. Eating carbohydrates can boost serotonin levels, a fact which may explain why SAD victims crave carbohydrates. The exposure to bright light appears to influence serotonin production, and to some extent, works the same way as antidepressant drugs.

As a result of more study over the past decade, the general consensus is that SAD, like other mood disorders may be initiated by biochemical disturbances. The role of melatonin and serotonin are vital to controlling mood, and appetite. Exposure to light seems to determine some of these cyclic patterns.

What is particularly fascinating is that the classic symptoms of SAD are strikingly similar to those of PMS, carbohydrate cravers, and obese individuals. These symptoms include: lethargy, over eating, weight gain, the inability to concentrate, and depression.[67] In all three of these disorders, the symptoms occurred only during certain time intervals; for SAD, during dark, winter months, for PMS, just prior to the menstrual period and for carbohydrate cravers, during the late afternoon or evening hours.

Peter S. Mueller, a psychiatrist at the Institute for Mental Health, after reviewing data, began experimenting with 2500 lux light to treat depressed women. Subsequently, eating habits of obese study groups were closely monitored at MIT's Clinical Research Center. It was discovered that carbohydrate cravers overeat only carbohydrates and do so only at certain times of the day. While calorie intake was normal at mealtime, snacking in the late afternoon or early evening dramatically increased caloric intake.

This same type of eating pattern was found in women suffering from PMS. Almost all of the snacks consumed were carbohydrates. Protein snacks were rarely selected. As mentioned in the Foods and Moods chapter, these carbohydrate cravings can be difficult to satiate, and frequently, the desire to eat may continue until inordinate amounts of food are consumed. Eating in attempt to elevate your mood is far different than eating to satisfy normal hunger.

This same type of cyclic eating is typical of people suffering from SAD. Finding the common denominator among these groups of people is vital to our understanding of any behavioral disorder. When carbohydrate cravers were given psychiatric evaluations, they were found to demonstrate a high susceptibility to depression. One SAD victim expressed, "I eat to combat a feeling of mental fatigue." What Mueller and others found was that exposing SAD patients to a few hours of sufficient light every morning could not only eliminate depression, but their carbohydrate craving as well. It has been suggested that obese individuals and women suffering from PMS may also be candidates for photo or light therapy.

Using supplemental light in the morning seems to be the most effective kind. Research has found that the decline of melatonin, which usually occurs early in the morning, is delayed in SAD sufferers. The serotonin connection links SAD, and PMS. In other words, decreased serotonin levels can make you feel depressed and can trigger a craving for carbohydrates.

Serotonin promoting drugs have a tendency to suppress carbohydrate snacking and relieve depression. For this reason, drugs that boost serotonin neurotransmission such as d-fenfluramine, femoxetine, fluoxetine, symelidine and fluvoxamine have a tendency to promote weight loss. On the other hand, drugs that clock serotonin action or antidepressants that affect other neurotransmitters instead of serotonin can create carbohydrate cravings and weight gain.

So what exactly is SAD then? The general consensus is that for many of us, our lifestyles increase our susceptibility to seasonal depression by decreasing our exposure to adequate light. Perhaps one of the reasons depression is much more prevalent during the twentieth century than previous time periods is that our ancestors had to spend a certain amount of time in the sun to survive. The very nature of our indoor jobs can predispose some of us to these types of mood disorders. While there is still much research needed on the subject, unquestionably, light affects our biochemistry.

LIGHT EXPOSURE AND VITAMIN D

Without ultra-violet light, our bodies cannot produce sufficient amounts of vitamin D. As a result, calcium cannot be adequately absorbed into the bones and teeth. While some foods provide vitamin D, studies have shown that these sources are not as biologically effective as the vitamin D produced in the skin from sunlight exposure. Even our dog, Emerson will find the only patch of sunlight we get in our northern exposure home and makes sure he gets his daily sunbath. Incidentally, there is some speculation that the presence of smog in urban areas can inhibit the efficiency of ultra violet light rays, impacting mood, and vitamin D absorbtion.

A study of elderly men living in a nursing home is Boston found that when isolated from natural daylight for seven weeks and exposed to only fluorescent or incandescent light, calcium absorption was significantly impaired due to a drop in vitamin D levels. It would be interesting to see if a drop in mood also corresponded to this sunlight deprivation. Again, many elderly people who are confined to poorly lit interiors suffer from serious depression. The availability of outdoor porches and verandas in convalescent homes has decreased over the last few decades. Sadly, most windows in professional care facilities don't even open.

LIGHT BOX THERAPY

Using light therapy to combat SAD involves a powerful light box of up to 10,000 lux which utilizes fluorescent tubes rather than full spectrum lighting. These boxes are designed for placement at a table and can be tilted to maximize exposure over the person, who can read or perform other tasks while being treated.

Ultra-violet rays are screened to prevent injury and reflected light is absorbed by the eyes. You don't have to use a sunscreen when using these boxes. The amount of ultra-violet light you'll get isn't enough to cause any degree of tanning. Full-spectrum light bulbs are used in these boxes. This light is closer to natural sunlight than fluorescent or regular light bulbs.

If you actually have SAD, you should start to see an improvement within the first few days of light therapy. If you're not sure you have SAD, discuss trying the box out on a trail basis before you invest the money to purchase one. There are over ten thousand of these light boxes in use today. Portable light dosage systems are also available.

The average light box costs between $350 and $400. If you think this is too expensive, consider the overall cost of prescription drugs and psychotherapy. Preliminary research has shown that these light boxes help up to 85 percent of people suffering from SAD. If you can't afford a light box, ask your doctor if he has one, or if one can be rented.

What about the possible value of light therapy for other forms of depression? Some psychiatrists have suggested that phototherapy may be of value in treating non-seasonal depression. There is evidence that exposing depressed individuals to bright light may be as effective in reducing some types of depression than antidepressant drugs.[68] More research is needed. The studies done by the Wurtmans certainly suggest that light may play a much more significant role in disorders such as PMS and obesity than previously thought.

In the meantime, if you suffer from any kind of depression, provide your environment with sufficient light and invest in a light box if you think it might help. Consider putting in a skylight too. Make your environment as light accessible as possible. Place reading chairs and worktops near windows. Keep your curtains drawn back or invest in lightweight shades or blinds that don't block out light. Don't clutter window sills or place furniture in front of light sources. Use light colored paints and upholstery and purchase track lighting that can be added to your existing ceiling light fixture. Keep your home well ventilated with fresh air and bring colorful plants and flowers into your environment.

For those who live in agreeable climates, make sure you get out in the sun every day for at least a couple of hours. Make sure you check with your doctor before initiating any kind of light therapy. There are certain eye conditions and skin disorders in which phototherapy should not be used.

RESOURCES:

National Organization for Seasonal Affective Disorder
P.O. Box 40133
Washington. D.C.
20016

National Depressive and Manic Depressive Association
730 Franklin, No. 501,
Chicago, Illinois
60610
800-826-3632

EXERCISE FOR DEPRESSION

*"The body is a test tube. You have to put in exactly
the right ingredients to get the best reaction out of it."*
Jack Youngblood

Understandably, if you're suffering from depression, exercising is the last thing you feel like doing. Depression has been described by some experts as a state of high energy turned inward. For this reason, trying to suppress or deny depression can only make it worse. If you think of depression as a form of negative energy, then the prospects of transforming that energy into movement can make more sense.

Some experts believe that depression can be a form of anger turned outside in. Marjorie Brooks, Ph.D. of Jefferson Medical College in Philadelphia says, "Low grade depression is found more often in women than in men. Some women may feel powerless at times, but instead of getting mad, they get depressed, As a result, they may constantly feel tired or have a chronic 'headachy' feeling."[69]

Releasing anger or frustration through exercise is highly recommended for its variety of beneficial effects. More and more research supports that fact that exercise is a powerful therapy against mood fluctuations. Robert S. Brown, Ph.D., M.D. and his colleagues at the University of Virginia have utilized a number of different physical activities to snap their patients out of depressive states. They believe, to some extent that the dramatic lack of movement that is so typical of a depressed person may in itself aggravate further depression.

When you're depressed, you want to withdraw, losing interest in practically everything. The depressed person is consumed with unhappy thoughts, that in some cases are so profound they actually incapacitate the body. Some doctors believe that if you sit and lay around too long, you may develope what is called a primary movement disorder, which always makes depression worse.

Numerous studies have proven that if you break out of lethargic behavior and force yourself to move, a more positive self-image will emerge. Even minor, very low impact exercise like walking around the block can create significant beneficial psychological changes according to Ronald Lawrence M.D., Ph.D., a California neurologist.

EXERCISE CAN EXORCISE THE DEMONS OF DEPRESSION

Dr. Andrew Weil, M.D. claims that he knows of no better method than aerobic exercise in the form of thirty minutes of continuous activity for at least five days a week for relieving symptoms of depression. What's even more encouraging, is that its hard to feel sad while your exercising. Dr. Russ Jaffe, Director of the Princeton Brain Bio Center maintains the "recent onset depression is hard to sustain with low impact aerobic exercise."[70] He goes on to suggest swimming, bicycling, cross country skiing, and even a brisk walk followed by a warm shower, followed by a cold shower are powerful weapons against depressive illness.

The psychological benefits of regular exercise cannot be overemphasized. All kinds of exercise can help you to become in tune with your body and its needs. While you're exercising, you can mediate and perhaps unravel some of the problems you must face. What's even more wonderful is that exercise can naturally do what drugs try to accomplish, which is to elevate certain brain amines that make us feel happier.

Most of us are aware of studies that show that after a certain amount of sustained exercise, brain endorphins are released which can create feeling of invigoration and well being. Marathon runners seem particularly susceptible to this type of "high" in which they experience euphoric altered states of consciousness. It is also true that aerobic exercise causes norepinephrine to be released in brain cells. By now, we're well aware that depression can be caused by a deficiency of norepinephrine. When you jog, your levels of this neurotransmitter increase, a phenomenon which lasts even after you stop.

In light of its connection to the biochemical makeup of the brain, exercise can be an effective tool for fighting depression. There's no question that exercising can help to lift your spirits. Learning to walk briskly every day or to jog at a moderate pace not only eases the blues, it provides a whole host of physical benefits as well. Vigorous regular exercise can help relive insomnia, poor appetite, irritability and anxiety, symptoms which usually accompany depression. It's also very inexpensive.

Two of the basic requirements for a healthy and happy life are fresh air and exercise, to which the benefit of sunlight exposure is also added. If we were smart, we would view exercise as crucial to our survival. Unfortunately, even when we feel relatively happy, its hard for us to make time to exercise. If we're depressed, we have to fight our way out of a force that can paralyze us.

Getting outdoors to exercise is the ideal scenario for anyone suffering from the "glums." Even on a overcast day, the light intensity is around 10,000 lux. For anyone suffering from a seasonal affective disorder, exercising for 30 minutes outdoors is the equivalent of a daily session of light therapy.[71]

Exercising outside can also raise the oxygen level of our cells which can directly impact how much physical and mental energy we generate. When we breathe deeply, we expedite the removal of carbon dioxide and other waste products from our systems. Remember, during states of depression, regional blood flow to brain tissue is usually decreased. Exercising does just the opposite. Some experts have claimed that it is virtually impossible to sustain a mental state of anger, depression or anxiety during and right after vigorous exercise. Some studies have shown that jogging for 30 minutes three times a week can be as effective or even more so that psychotherapy sessions. Numerous women have passionately related how regular exercise literally saved them from an emotional crisis experienced during menopause.

An added bonus of exercise, and we could go on forever, is that when we increase our heart rate and energy is expended, more calories are burned, weight is lost and sudden drops in blood sugar are usually prevented. In other words, exercising can help stem sudden carbohydrate cravings due to low blood sugar.

If you've felt low for an extended period of time, you know how many aches and pains have accompanied the depression. Regular exercise can help to alleviate stiff muscles and joints and can boost the digestive system so elimination is more efficient. When you exercise, you sleep better, breathe easier, and think clearer.

Dr. John Greist who has written a paper entitled, "Running Out of Depression" conducted a study of 28 depressed patients and found that those patients who ran controlled their depression much better than those who were treated with psychotherapy. Even if you can only get out three days a week, the emotional benefits of regular exercise cannot be overstated.

If depression can be treated with physical activity, it only stands to reason that a lack of physical activity might bring it on. Depression may result if you lead a sedentary life. Are you physically immobile? Inactivity and excessive confinement punish the human body, both mentally and physically. We were not meant to sit around and loafe.

MAKE EXERCISE WORK FOR YOU AS A POWERFUL ANTIDEPRESSANT

Decide now to make regular exercise a part of your life. Start slow and easy. Choose the time of the day that feels the most natural and affords you the best opportunity for success. Don't pick 4:00 AM to go running. While early morning may be the ideal time, make sure you're a morning person. Exercising after work or before dinner is just as good. Exercising with a companion is recommended and making it as pleasant as possible is a plus. Using music to enhance your exercise is particularly beneficial as it can energize your body and elevate your mood. Scientific studies have proven that music makes exercise more enjoyable and easier to accomplish.

You might want to incorporate jogging or walking as your main mode of transportation. During your lunch break, get out of the office and eat lunch outside. Walk around the block before you return to work. If you can find a walking companion, that's great, but walking alone can also have its benefits. Walk a dog, walk where and when it's safe, and walk consistently. Establish a routine. Do it for your physical, emotional and spiritual well being.

Brisk walking is especially good. Let's face it, the aging process itself can be depressing and walking is a great anti-aging defense. If you walk briskly for at least 15 to 30 minutes a day, you can expect to feel a considerable mental lift. Brisk walking or jogging can enable you to take control of your depression. It's a natural prescription for low moods that is based on sound scientific data.

When you jog or walk briskly, epinephrine, norepinephrine, serotonin and endorphins are all increased. In many depressed individuals, norepinephrine which is measured by detecting a substance called MHPG is decreased. Exercising causes MHPG levels to rise. As a result of this elevated level of norepinephrine, depressed can be reversed and synaptic transmission in the brain stimulated. Exercise acts as a "wake up" call to your brain. Moreover, the serotonin connection, which keeps popping up throughout every section of this book, involves exercising as well. Positron emission scans have revealed that during exercise, the right part of the brain is activated resulting in fantasizing, uncluttered thinking or a state of mental awareness. In addition to this, serotonin, which determines mood, rises. As a result, you feel happier.

Become aware of your body and its connection with your state of mind. Something as benign as sitting around can have devastating physical and mental effects. Some scientists believe that even something as seemingly insignificant as your posture can cause depression. Stand straight, breathe deeply, carry yourself with pride, and exercise on a regular basis.

Dr. Kenneth Cooper relates, "Many days when I run several miles, I have a much greater awareness of my body than ever had before. Sometimes, at the end of a good run, my body seems to be working like a well-oiled machine. I may start the run in a fragmented emotional state, with many concerns and worries about various things, but by the end of such a run, I feel whole. My mind and my body become one."[72] Before you begin to exercise, remember that no fitness program can be truly successful if you don't utilize the powers of the mind as well as the body. You must want to be healthy. Desire is everything.

By now, it should be clearly understood that exercise can act as a powerful antidote to depression. Vigorous workouts can not only initiate chemical reactions that elevate mood, they can also give you a sense of purpose and control and that helps dispel gloomy outlooks. The benefits of regular exercise are staggering to say the least. To the person who suffers from depression, exercise should be viewed as nothing short of life-saving.

UNRECOGNIZED CAUSES
OF DEPRESSION

*"Discovery consists in seeing what everybody has seen
and thinking what nobody has thought."*

Albert Szent-Gyorgyi

Recently, some doctors have discovered what natural medicine has advocated for centuries; that people suffering from psychiatric illnesses frequently have a number of physical problems as well. In fact, many people who are depressed are reacting to a physiological stressor, rather than a psychological one. In other words, virtually any illness or disruption in our biology can precipitate feeling "blue." Some of the more prevalent of these are: excessive dieting, yeast infections, food intolerances, allergies, malnutrition and hormonal imbalances. Not only can these disorders attend depressive illness, in many cases they are the major cause of its development.

One psychiatrist relates:

"After my training, I found there were patients who weren't responding quickly enough to psychotherapy. I wanted to see if there was another approach. I began using orthomolecular techniques, which were not accepted in regular psychiatric circles. The more I got into it, the more I realized the importance of clinical nutrition and how much the endocrine system affects thoughts and moods. Not only can our minds cause illness, but physical illnesses can produce systemic imbalances that may lead to profound emotional and mental changes. Many people who come to me with psychiatric symptoms have physical problems, like allergies, viral infections, malnutrition, and endocrine disorders. Once we treat these conditions, the psychological symptoms clear up."[73]

The reverse of this premise is also true: feeling down can trigger a number of physical changes that can increase our vulnerability to disease. It is a well documented fact that depressive behavior can impair the immune system, making its victims susceptible to a wide variety of ailments.

Dr. Marvin Stein of the Mt. Sinai School of Medicine at the City University of New York and his colleagues studied a group of widowers soon after they had lost their wives and found a decrease in T and B cell activity. B and T cells are a vital part of our immune systems. For this reason, disorders like Chronic Fatigue Syndrome, which is believed to be caused by the Epstein-Barr virus can be linked to depression, either as a causal effect or as a result of.

Similar testing has shown that depressed people have significantly poorer DNA or genetic repair of their cells. Doctors at Ohio State University discovered that the cells of people who suffered from mood disorders which were exposed to radiation, regenerated at a slower rate. Some possible ramifications of these findings include the possibility that emotional stress may contribute to the incidence of cancer by causing abnormal cell development or by weakening the bodies defense system against carcinogen exposure.[74]

Unquestionably, a relationship between the severity of depression and a suppression of the immune system exists. Doctors have also found that when depression subsides, T and B cell production increases. This particular phenomenon is not restricted to the human animal alone. Studies done with dogs showed similar results. A dog who was used to being loved and affectionately petted was left completely alone for an extended period of time. He was given plenty of nutritious food and an ample water supply, but was denied physical contact. At periodic intervals, his bone marrow was checked for changes. After a couple of weeks, the dog acted depressed and changes in his white and red blood cell count occurred. In essence, his immune system was compromised, and it was all due to a lack of love and attention.

Tests done at George Washington University of cancer patients found that those who engaged in regular relaxation exercises and used creative imagery to foster feelings of well being and health experienced positive changes in their immune systems. The production of antibodies, lymphocytes and interleukin-2 cells increased in proportion to the practice of stress relieving exercise and creative mental imagery.[75]

The message here is clear. If we get depressed for what ever reason, our ability to fight disease is inhibited. The reverse can also be true, which brings up a whole host of possible relationships between biological impairments and mental health. Everything from food allergies to fungal infections may be intrinsically linked to our emotional status.

Several illnesses can cause you to feel depressed and include: anemia, hypothyroidism, candida, multiple sclerosis, and colon disorders. In addition, a vast number of drugs and environmental toxins can produce the same results. It may well be that your depression stems from one of these factors. You need to find out.

Education is the key. You may be surprised at what you learn. So many of us who suffer from unexplained depression assume that we possess some inherent flaw in our characters. Some of us may view our depression as a kind of punishment for not measuring up. How would you feel if you discovered the real culprit was a chronic yeast infections, your weight loss plan, an inactive thyroid or a hidden food allergy? The good news is that when you treat any of these disorders including depression with natural medicine, you will inevitably improve your overall health as well.

Listed below are medical conditions that may cause depression:

- AIDS
- ADDISON'S DISEASE
- CANCER
- CHRONIC FATIGUE SYNDROME
- CUSHING'S DISEASE
- DEMENTIAS (INCLUDING ALZHEIMER'S DISEASE)
- ENDOCRINE DISORDERS SUCH AS HYPOTHYROIDISM
- EPILEPSY (TEMPORAL LOBE)
- FOOD ALLERGIES
- HUNTINGTON'S DISEASE
- HYPOGLYCEMIA
- INFLUENZA
- LUPUS ERYTHEMATOSUS, SYSTEMIC
- MONONUCLEOSIS
- MULTIPLE SCLEROSIS
- PERNICOUS ANEMIA
- PORPHYRIA, INTERMITTENT
- STROKE
- SYPHILLIS
- VITAMIN DEFICIENCIES (ESPECIALLY FOLIC ACID, VITAMIN B-6 AND B-12)
- YEAST INFECTIONS

Let's look into some of the more common and unrecognized biological causes of depression. We will address those physical conditions which routinely predispose a person to depression. In each and every instance, the delicate balance of the brain's neurochemistry is altered.

DIETING, EATING DISORDERS AND DEPRESSION

"Food is fun and sound nutrition need not diminish the pleasure. More than anything else, it's the nonsense of nutrition...the unreasonable food fears and unnecessary prohibitions ...that takes the joy out of eating...Without an adequate amount and proper balance of nutrients, you are simply not going to live as long or as healthily, look as good, or work as hard as you are genetically programmed to do."

Paul Saltman, Ph.D.
The California Nutrition Book

The food and mood connection is strongly evidenced in our pervasive obsession with weight control in this country. Dangerous dieting and a variety of devastating eating disorders can significantly contribute to depressive illness, especially among young women. Consistently going off and on diets, the use of diet pills, and eating disorders like bulimia and anorexia exact an enormous emotional and mental toll on our society. Being overweight has been traditionally associated with depressive illness, however, recently, a new slant on the problem has emerged.

For years, psychiatrists assumed that the reason that overweight people seemed more vulnerable to depressive illness centered around their dissatisfaction with how they looked. New research has found that it is dieting, not the extra weight, which causes moods to plummet.

The yo yo syndrome of losing and gaining weight, and the constant nutritional stressors of dieting directly impact the incidence of depression. It's not surprising to learn that yet another piece of evidence supporting the very real effect of food on mood has recently surfaced. Unfortunately, dieting is a way of life in our country.

DIETING: *A LEADING DOCUMENTED CAUSE OF DEPRESSION*

The Journal of Health and Social Behavior reports that researchers asked over 2,000 men and women between the ages of 18 to 90 to complete a standard checklist designed to detect symptoms of depression. The questionnaire also surveyed their nutritional and exercise habits, their weight, height, etc. The study concluded that dieting was the leading cause of depression in overweight people.[76]

Cutting calories puts much more stress on mental outlook than previously assumed. After looking at the stats, researchers strongly recommended that if you're overweight, burn more calories rather than eliminate them. Making exercise a regular part of lifestyle was seen as the best alternative for overweight individuals. "...for mental health, the overweight would be best served by increasing their exercise levels rather than dieting, if they want to lose weight."[77]

CARBOHYDRATE DEPLETION AND LOW MOODS

Any of us who have dieted, and who hasn't, would agree that most diets are overly restrictive and usually require the elimination of so many of the foods we are accustomed to eating. The carbohydrate restrictive diets would be particularly detrimental to mood, as we discussed in a earlier section.

Eating healthfully rarely goes hand and hand with dieting. All too often, when we diet, we go without sufficient nutrients assuming that we have to in order to lose weight. Just feeling deprived can make us moody and irritable, not to mention the physiological reactions which can initiate low serotonin levels or vitamin and mineral depletion. This same study found that eating healthily, which involved following a low-fat not no-fat diet that was high in complex carbohydrates and fresh fruits and vegetables did not promote depression.

Using diet aids, such as appetite suppressants can also result in mood alteration. The overwhelming majority of dieters and diet pill abusers are young females. A study done at the University of San Francisco found that of 500 girls, almost half of those who were only nine years old and 80 percent of those ages ten and eleven were dieting.[78] The enormous number of these girls who excessively diet and use over-the-counter appetite suppressants is cause for considerable concern.

DIET PILLS, PPA AND DEPRESSION

Vivian Hanson Meechan, president of the National Association of Anorexia Nervosa and Associated Disorders said, "Diet pills containing the drug phenylpropanolamine or PPA, pose a very serious health risk to adolescents."[79] This is not the first time we've brought up the negative effects of PPA on mood. She went on to disclose that a minimum of one out of every ten teenagers engages in dangerous eating practices which include starvation diets, binge eating, vomiting, abusing laxative and diuretics and taking diet pills.

According to some biopsychiatrists, the incredible amount of calories consumed by bulimics and their compulsive, frenzied eating followed by deliberate vomiting is a physically induced behavior. In other words, a disturbance in brain chemistry may be the primary causal factor of this type of eating disorder. Women who suffer from bulimia are more likely to have other psychological problems. Depression is one of the most common of these.

Once again, the question of which came first, the depression or the bulimia remains unanswered. Today, it is common to treat bulimia with antidepressants, which serves to confirm the link between brain chemistry and the behavior. Even if you are a bulimic who is not depressed, taking antidepressants seems to help control the eating disorder. The role of neurotransmitters, especially serotonin and norepinephrine must be considered here.

DIETING CAN DEPLETE SEROTONIN

Unquestionably, certain changes in brain chemistry can result from eating disorders. In addition, starvation lowers supplies of norepinephrine which can create mental lethargy and indifference. Bulimics commonly have lower than normal levels of serotonin also. It's beginning to get a little redundant at this point, but it must be reiterated once again; serotonin deficiencies are associated with depression. Interestingly, as we discussed in the Food and Sugar section, if you are low in serotonin, you constantly reach for carbohydrates in excessive amounts. The low serotonin levels of bulimics may also help to explain their uncontrollable binging, which often targets carbohydrate foods.

This same phenomenon explains why dieting is so hard for most of us. The most common reason for abandoning a diet is dealing with the serotonin depletion we experience. The classic symptoms of dieting, which included, irritability, depression, moodiness, and nervousness can be the direct result of a serotonin deficiency, created by a lack of carbohydrates. What usually happens is that we stick to a diet until we absolutely can't stand it, and then we go on a carbohydrate rampage, eating anything and everything in sight. Consequently we may feel guilty, but our initial mood will probably elevate and our anxiety will go down. This kind of eating, however, eventually results in more weight gain, and so the cycle keeps repeating itself over and over. The Wurtman study we referred to in earlier sections has concluded that diets that are too carbohydrate restricted will ultimately fail because they are not "brain friendly."

The answer then to this deplorable dilemma is to manage your carbohydrate intake and to eat the right things at the right time. Raw vegetables, fruits, and complex carbohydrates like certain low fat cereals etc, should be eaten instead of cookies, pies, and chips. To try to deny yourself carbohydrates when you crave them is futile. It's much better to re-design your food options, eat heartily and exercise.

In regards to the value of dieting, perhaps we need to re-assess our goals. The physiology of the brain directly bears on how and what you eat. Eating and mood are closely connected and must be understood in order to understand weight gain and weight loss.

If serotonin levels are so crucial to both depression and carbohydrate craving, amino acid and vitamin therapy may be extremely valuable in helping to control neurotransmitters levels, which can propel us into uncontrolled eating and depressive illness.

FOOD ALLERGIES AND MOOD DISORDERS

"One man's meat is another man's poison."

Lucretius, first century B.C. poet

When it comes to the subject of food allergies, the above quote seems especially appropriate. There is plenty of speculation and some compelling evidence that the relationship between food and behavior is a very real one. Moreover, what can be eaten by one person without any detrimental results, can cause another to feel and act lousy. Several prominent physicians have linked food allergies to depression not to mention migraines, schizophrenia, arthritis, obesity and eczema. Generally speaking, however, conventional medicine refutes the connection.

Naturally, over the past several years, the subject of food allergies has spawned substantial controversy. Like hypoglycemia, their existence is questioned by some physicians. The entire notion of food sensitivities causing behavioral or mood disorders has received a cool reception within the scientific community. Concerning this all too familiar reluctance to accept anything which has eluded the medical books, Michel de Montaigne puts it well:

"Whenever a new discovery is reported to the scientific world, they say first, 'it is probably not true.' Thereafter, when the truth of the new proposition has been demonstrated beyond question, they say, 'Yes, it may be true, but it is not important.' Finally, when sufficient time has elapsed to fully evidence its importance they say, 'Yes, surely it is important, but it is no longer new.'"[80]

Whether accepted or not, sensitivities to food substances do in fact exist and are unfortunately, on the rise. Several theories exist which attempt to explain the proliferation of food allergies. No doubt, factors such as breathing polluted air, ingesting hidden chemical and toxic metals in food and water, stress, and poor dietary habits have contributed to the development of these hypersensitivities.

HOW DO YOU DEFINE A FOOD ALLERGY?

What is a food allergy exactly? An intolerance to certain foods does not bring on the same kind of symptoms we normally associate with allergies; watery eyes, sneezing, wheezing, hives, runny nose etc. A food allergy is based on some type of malfunction, probably digestive in nature that has not been fully explained to date. Because of this reason, some scientists are slow to recognize its existence, nevertheless, its symptoms and its obvious effect on certain individuals cannot be ignored. What we eat can and does affect how we act.

Many nutritionists wholeheartedly accept the fact that food allergies frequently cause hyperkinetic behavior in children. In these instances, children with Attention Deficit Disorder are immediately taken off of sugar, wheat and chemical additives. There is substantial evidence that hyperactivity is related to what one eats. In other words, the metabolic role of diet in a sensitive person can play havoc with brain biochemistry.

Elisa Lotter Ph.D. relates the story of Henry, who at age 17 had been on tranquilizers, electric shock treatments and psychotherapy for several years with no significant improvement. He was subsequently placed on a strict fast in which he was given only spring water. After 4 days, he experienced a complete reversal of symptoms, until the 5th day, in which he was given a meal consisting of only wheat. Within an hour, he began to experience negative, paranoid thoughts. Further testing confirmed that when certain foods were withheld from Henry, his symptoms disappeared; when they were added, he became mentally disturbed once again.[81]

Likewise, Doctors Philpott and Kalita in their book *Brain Allergies*, discuss the very significant mental impact that dairy products and cereal grains have in some schizophrenics. The implication here is that hidden food sensitivities and intolerances may be responsible for a number of emotional disorders in certain susceptible people.

The very nature of what we eat is often unknown to us. In other words, we very willingly open microwaveable dinners, brightly colored boxes, and bags and gladly ingest a number of mystery ingredients and chemicals. Marshall Mandell, M.D. who has written two books and numerous scientific papers on the subject of food intolerance discusses the fact that when man tampers with natural food substances they can become contaminants rather than nutrients to the body. He states: "Furthermore, contemporary mass-production strips food of many valuable nutrients that, were they left intact, would provide protective benefits."[82] The question remains; can eating a doughnut and a glass of milk make you feel sad?

Apparently, there are several ways in which a food allergy can trigger a change in mood. During an allergic reaction, the body leaks histamine from the capillaries, which can cause edema or swelling around them. This is well understood by those who suffer from pollen allergies. If you have hay fever, your sinuses swell and you can't breath through your nose. Dr. Mandell believes that the same reaction can take place in brain cells when you eat a culprit food, causing a disruption in brain chemistry.

In addition, in the same way that muscle spasms cause the bronchiole tubes to constrict during an allergic asthma attack, he proposes that similar spasms in the small arteries of the brain can reduce the flow of glucose, oxygen and other nutrients to brain tissue. Both of these scenarios would naturally precipitate a change in behavior or mood. Regardless of its mechanisms, sensitivities to certain foods can make us feel mentally and physically depressed. This is the reason why some people feel unusually good when they fast.

If you have allergies to certain foods, you won't just experience a change in mood. In fact, like the role of sugar in hypoglycemia, you may be initially stimulated by eating a food you are allergic to. Symptoms are frequently delayed and therefore, misdiagnosed.

SYMPTOMS OF FOOD SENSITIVITIES

Multiple symptoms are typical of food intolerances and should be watched for. Billy Casper, famous for his golfing, complained for years of weight gain, stomach aliments, sinus congestion, backaches, headaches and a bad temper. Apparently, after some investigation and testing, he was found to be food sensitive to beet sugar, lamb, apples, pork, eggs, citrus fruit, wheat and any fruits or vegetables fertilized with nitrates or sprayed with chemicals. Billy Casper changed his lifestyle and his diet, and his health, particularly his moods significantly improved.[83] The most common symptoms in adults of a food allergy are depression, headaches and fatigue. Mood changes can range from mild forms of anxiety to feeling seriously depressed. Manic outbursts of uncontrollable anger are also possible. The relationship between food allergies and schizophrenia may be profound one for some patients. The notion that something you ate is driving you wild is particularly applicable here.

Two types of reactions can occur if you eat something you are sensitive to. Initially, there can be an immediate reaction characterized by symptoms which quickly occur and are easy to recognize. If you eat shrimp and break out in hives, or develop an unusual headache etc. you know the shrimp is probably responsible. It's the second type of reaction to a food which is more difficult to identify because it may not occur for a day or two. If you ate a large meal and various foods on Sunday, you may feel overly fatigued, lethargic and depressed on Tuesday. In these cases, connecting your symptoms with a meal you ate a couple of days ago is unlikely. Obviously, the link is difficult to make.

Several medical journals in the 1980's published articles which proposed that delayed food allergies caused nearly all cases of migraine headaches. In addition, reports in the *Journal of Arthritis and Rheumatism* disclosed that many cases of rheumatoid and osteoarthritis cleared up when certain offending foods were removed from the diet.[84]

For this reason, perhaps calling this phenomenon a food allergy is not totally accurate because the same kind of immune processes that occur with a typical allergy are not found in these situations. To make matters worse, symptoms of a food allergy can mimic other conditions.

HYPOGLYCEMIA AND FOOD INTOLERANCE

Because the symptoms are so similar, it is easy to mistake a food allergy for hypoglycemia. Both are directly related to an improper diet and share the same type of relationship with meals. In addition, a food allergy can cause an abnormal insulin response, which could show up as hypoglycemia on a glucose tolerance test. What is really fascinating is that both hypoglycemia and food allergies can often be controlled by restricting highly refined carbohydrates and some grains such as wheat.[85]

Dr. Mandell's study of 200 hospitalized schizophrenics found that 65 percent were sensitive to wheat products and 50 percent to milk and corn products.[86] He also found that the most frequently craved and eaten foods continually resulted in the worst symptoms. In addition, the amount of a food and how often it was eaten played a significant role. In other words, a certain food eaten once a week may be tolerated by the body, however, if it is eaten every day, it may cause symptoms to develop.

HOW DO YOU BECOME FOOD ALLERGIC AND WHAT SHOULD YOU DO?

How does one develop a food allergy? Interestingly, you can become sensitive to the same food that you have spent years overeating. The theory here is that eventually, this particular food may become dangerous to the body because it is perceived as an allergen, just like pollen. What is even more interesting about the research done on food allergies is that frequently, the body craves the very food that causes it to feel ill. If you stop eating a certain food you have consumed for years, you can develop a set of symptoms that are not relieved until you eat that particular food again. Talk about a vicious cycle.

Foods which are commonly associated with allergic reactions include: cow's milk products, wheat, eggs, yeast, corn, soy, cane sugar, dyes and preservatives. It is not uncommon to also become allergic to beef, chicken, lettuce, artificial sweeteners and tobacco. There has been some speculation that even the water we consume may cause allergic reactions in some people. For this reason, if you find that you are food sensitive, use bottled water rather than chlorinated of fluoridated supplies.

Discovering your "culprit" foods is a formidable task. If you are suffering from inexplicable symptoms which include depression, anxiety, uncontrolled crying, chronic fatigue or diarrhea, you may want to eliminate suspect foods from your diet for a period of two weeks. Keep in mind, that you might not feel all that great when you stop eating these foods as the body goes into a kind of withdrawal. Some experts recommend starting with a 24 hour fast first and assessing how you feel.

After the two weeks is over, begin to reintroduce these foods, one at a time every 48 hours in large quantities and watch yourself closely for any symptoms. If you suffer from asthma or severe emotional disorders, do not attempt this test alone. Consult a specialist. Food allergy testing is also available. Remember that if you suspect that corn is a culprit, you must also eliminate corn oil, corn syrup and corn starch. These are ingredients commonly found in packaged foods.

Learn to read all labels. Assessing something as elusive as food allergies takes a great deal of nutritional detective work. When all is said and done, if you suspect that certain foods are causing you to feel depressed, look for evidence of food addiction in cravings and over eating and other physical symptoms including: morning headaches, fatigue and fluctuations in weight.

Supplementing your diet with an adequate supply of vitamin C and specific bioflavonoids (quercetin, rutin, hesperidin, pycnogenol and catechin) can help to facilitate detoxification reactions which occur from a food allergy. Bioflavonoids can work to stabilize mast cells in the bowel that release histamine when triggered by the presence of an allergen.

In certain parts of the country, a blood test to measure the presence of the immunoglobulin G, may also help to determine if you have a food allergy. This test is called the IgE-IgG RAST test or the ELISA/ACT test. Skin testing for food allergies is highly ineffective, and the reliability of pendulum swings or electro-acupuncture is still questionable. The blood test can conclusively show if you have an immune system reaction to certain foods. If you are interested in pursuing this avenue contact:

Quantum Analytical Laboratory
38 D Anna Cade Road
Rockwell, Texas 75087
214-771-4422

The availability of the Cytotoxic test has also made it possible to investigate and discover food sensitivities with greater accuracy and ease. This particular test must be performed by a qualified technician. Bear in mind that the test in never 100% accurate.

In assessing foods that can cause a sensitivity in numerous individuals, gluten comes out at the top of the list. An intolerance to gluten, even a mild one has been cited as a plausible cause of depression. Dr. Alan Gaby M.D. states that gluten intolerance, which refers to a sensitivity to wheat, oats, barley and rye, may be much more common than previously assumed.[87] In this particular type of food sensitivity, a lack of vitamin B-6 can result which can cause a depressed mental state.

FOOD ALLERGIES AND MOOD DISORDERS

Again, it must be emphasized that the possibility that a food allergy may be causing you to feel melancholy is rarely pursued by physicians. Dr. Harvey Ross M.D. puts it this way: "One major flaw of modern psychiatry is the exclusive pursuit of psychotherapy or drug therapy for patients who lack energy and clear thinking. Such problems often have nutritional causes, and when treated, facilitate psychotherapy tremendously or even eliminate the need for it...to unravel problems effectively, it is necessary to explore how and what a person eats, not just his family history and potentially significant emotional events."[88]

Effective treatment of any food sensitivity depends on the total elimination of the targeted food. If you eliminate suspect foods, you should feel better within a few weeks. Dr. Ross believes that after abstaining from these foods for several months, they may be slowly re-introduced into the diet as long as they are only eaten occasionally.

When evaluating the viability of a relationship between depression and allergies it must be remembered that what we eat in combination with what we breathe, drink and the very nature of our environments and personal relationships creates a synergistic effect on our mental and physical health.

BOWEL DISORDERS AND DEPRESSION

". . . many degenerative diseases are brought about by toxins generated in the large bowel. Bacterial flora imbalance, putrefaction, of undigested foods, parasitic and yeast infections may be at the bottom (excuse the pun) of many diseases."

Zolton P. Rona, M.D., MSc.

What goes on way down there in your intestines may seem totally unrelated to something like your mental attitude. If the facts in this book have done nothing else, they have demonstrated the intrinsic and fragile interconnection between all body systems. In other words, no organ is an island. The condition of the colon can be a predictor of health, and its condition is directly dependent on what we put in our mouths.

The idea of intestinal toxemia is based on the belief that the type of diet you eat determines the kind of bacteria found in your intestines. If you eat a lot of complex carbohydrates and little protein, your intestinal flora will primarily consists of bacteria that breakdown carbohydrates.

On the other hand, if your diet is high in protein and low in carbohydrates, intestinal bacteria will be of the proteolytic type which are designed to break down proteins or to decompose them. What is of interest to us at this point is that some scientists believe that this type of bacteria can transform amino acids which come from protein into powerful toxins.

Two amino acids in question are tryptophan and tyrosine, these should sound familiar by now. If you eat 94 grams of protein per day, which is the amount eaten by a large number of Americans, this protein can remain in the intestines too long. The fact that most of us eat low fiber diets potentiates this scenario as well. As a result, adverse chemical reactions can occur. In laymen's terms, eating a lot of meat can create delayed elimination. Consequently, poisons can form in the colon.

TYROSINE AND TRYPTOPAHN IN THE COLON: HIGH PROTEIN DIETS ARE NOT GOOD FOR THE HUMAN BODY

Tyrosine is converted to phenol and tryptophan to indole and skatole in the bowel. All of these by-products are considered toxic and are believed to re-enter the bloodstream to some extent. When this happens, the liver kicks in to detoxify them. Unfortunately, phenol can elude the filtering processes of the liver and may continue to circulate in the bloodstream.

It is the presence of phenol which some experts believe is responsible for a whole host of ailments ranging from allergies to arthritis to cancer, to back pain and mental illness. This particular phenomenon is referred to as autointoxication and is gaining more and more credibility among medical doctors.

Mainstream medicine has finally accepted the notion that eating too much protein is bad for human beings. A fact that was taught to doctors decades ago by respected medical colleagues. A paper read at the annual meeting of the American Medical Association in 1917 reported 517 cases of mental symptoms which were relieved by eliminating intestinal toxemia.[89]

In 1962, the same subject was addressed regarding schizophrenia and indole metabolism. Some of the mental symptoms listed at the 1917 medical convention from overeating meat were nervousness, fatigue, and general wretchedness, a particularly good way to describe depression itself.

We now know that a high protein diet aggravates colon disease. Eating a diet rich in complex carbohydrates and low in protein is praised as the ultimate health promoter. Eating this way results in a decrease of proteolytic bacteria which are responsible for the putrefaction which is created in our intestines.

How many Americans suffer from chronic gas, constipation and other digestive upsets caused by intestinal toxemia? Too many. Like the inordinate amounts of white sugar we ingest as a society, the excess availability of protein is not naturally accepted by our systems. To put it simply, we were not designed to dine on steak every night.

We should be eating 50 grams or protein per day rather than the typical 94. Some health care experts, recommend taking that down even further to 25 or 30 grams per day if you're not a child, pregnant, or nursing. The rampant over-consumption of meat in our country has contributed to a vast number of colon diseases. When the colon is compromised, overall health is jeopardized.

Remember also, that when it comes to maintaining healthy intestinal bacteria, we may be sabotaging ourselves. Many Americans routinely take antibiotics for everything from a cold to a hangnail. This glut of flora killing chemicals in the form of antibiotics may be adversely affecting thousands of people without their knowledge. Antibiotics can save lives and routinely do. There is no denying the fact, however, that they are grossly over-prescribed. It is not uncommon to see people who have been on antibiotic therapy for extended periods of time feeling lethargic or generally unwell. Friendly bacteria lost through antibiotics must be replaced. How many of us do that?

POOR NUTRIENT ABSORPTION IN THE COLON AND VITAMIN B DEPLETION

Evidence suggests that people who suffer from some bowel disorders related to food intolerance may be victims of vitamin B-6 deficiencies due to the nature of the disease. This fact has led certain doctors to believe that people with malabsorption problems may be more prone to depression. The relationship of food allergies plays a role here also. Being sensitive to certain grains is also typical of a number of colon disorders.

Celiac disease is caused by a food intolerance to any grain which contains gluten or gluten-like substances. The disease progressively causes the destruction of the surface of the small bowel, where nutrients are absorbed. Anytime a person with this disease eats a food they can't tolerate, more colon cell destruction occurs.

Depression is common to people suffering from celiac disease and various studies have linked this depression with a lack of vitamin B-6. They have found that treating the depression with vitamin B-6 supplements was quite successful. There are several implications here that should be considered.

Number one: the health of the colon and the functions that it provides can be linked not only with physical disorders, but mental ones as well.

Number two: how many of us suffer from hidden intolerances to certain foods like milk or wheat, which may be impairing our ability to absorb nutrients essential to maintaining good emotional and mental health?

If you suffer from chronic constipation or diarrhea, irritable bowel syndrome, spastic colon or colitis, you may be a candidate for depression. Turn your attention to your diet and eliminate culprit foods. Put white flour, white sugar, caffeine and alcohol at the top of your list. Wheat, and dairy products are also common offenders.

When the bowel is irritated or sluggish, it can be assumed that the effectiveness of nutrient absorption will be impaired to some extent. If this occurs over an extended period of time, deficiencies will occur. As previously established, a lack of the B vitamins can profoundly affect mental outlook. Irritable bowel syndrome and other colon related ailments are extremely common in the United States. Perhaps the epidemic proportions of depression experienced in this country are due, to some extent, to the high prevalence of colon disease. The typical American diet which is high in animal fat, dairy products and refined carbohydrates perpetuates colon disorders. In addition, this type of diet can also promote constipation, which may also play a significant role in determining emotional health and stability.

WHAT CONSTITUTES CONSTIPATION?

While much controversy exists on how often a healthy colon should eliminate waste, it is generally accepted that bowel movements should occur every 12 to 18 hours. For years, we've associated a grumpy disposition with constipation. In reality, prolonged constipation can be a contributing factor to depressed mental states.

Again, designing a diet that is high in legumes, raw fruits and vegetables, fiber and plenty of pure water can prevent constipation. We take more laxatives in this country than any other country in the world. This fact should serve as a wake up call. It testifies to the sad fact that our dietary habits tax our bodies rather than sustain them. Constipation is not a normal condition. Being continually constipated can significantly taint the way we view life and its challenges, not to mention our energy status. Additionally, keeping our intestinal flora healthy is also vital.

HORMONES AND DEPRESSION:

"It would seem that our glands effect control far above proportion to their size, and this is true. It is also true, however, that the glands have their master, probably the most remarkable creation in all of life's miracles — the human brain."

Dr. Bernard Jensen, Ph.D.

Twice as many women as men get depressed. Women who have just had a baby, women on the pill and postmenopausal women are prime candidates for depression. You don't have to be rocket scientist to figure out that hormonal imbalances cause depression. Obviously, pregnancy and delivery affect neurotransmitter production in the brain. In addition, studies reported in the *British Medical Journal* show that women who suffer from postmenopausal depression and younger women who suffer from depression prior to their periods have impaired tryptophan metabolism.

POSTPARTUM DEPRESSION, VITAMIN B AND FOLATE DEFICIENCIES

18 women who were depressed were tested for blood levels of tryptophan the week after they had given birth. Doctors discovered that those who were the most severely depressed had the lowest tryptophan levels.[90] Postpartum depression is the perfect example of a mental disorder caused by brain biochemistry. Zoltan P. Rona MD. states that researchers have shown that this type of depression may be due to a lack of B-complex vitamins, calcium and magnesium. Rona goes on to emphasize that medical literature cites several cases of postpartum depression that were essentially cured in a week by using high folic acid supplementation and vitamin B-12 injections.[91]

The American Journal of Obstetrics and Gynecology relates a case in which a woman suffered from an unusually serious case of postpartum depression. She became progressively worse during the weeks following the birth of her baby. Her emotional stability deteriorated to the point where she felt she might even harm herself or her new baby. She was hospitalized in two different psychiatric institutions and received shock treatments and various drugs. She showed no significant improvement and even tried to commit suicide three times.

Eventually her folate levels were tested and they were so low that one was labeled "undetectable." She began receiving five milligrams of folic acid twice a day, which is considered a mega-therapeutic dose. After ten days, she experienced a complete turn around. She was discharged and told to take one milligram of oral folic acid every day.[92] Supplementation with folic acid is considered safe for most dosages. The RDA for folic acid is set at 400 mcg for pregnant women, an amount considered pathetically low by a number of doctors.

PMS: A NUTRIENT DEFICIENCY DISORDER?

It is vital to stop here and emphasize again that most of us believe that we are eating right and getting enough vitamins and minerals. For many individuals, however, RDA dosages are not high enough. When you're dealing with the therapeutic use of minerals, amino acids and vitamins, a different approach to these nutrients is required. When it comes to counteracting hormonal stress, you have to go well beyond the RDA. Taking 50 milligrams of vitamin B-6 daily according to Dr. Alan Gaby, M.D. can significantly control the low moods and other symptoms that accompany PMS. This is 25 times the RDA for vitamin B-6.

Guy Abraham, M.D. believes that malnutrition and stress underpin PMS. He strongly recommends that women should avoid caffeine, sugar, nicotine, alcohol, salt, fatty or fried foods and excess dairy products. He advises a diet based on plenty of fresh fruits and vegetables, lean meats, legumes and whole grains. Where have we heard that before? What we haven't heard before is that red meats and dairy products may contain estrogen, which only serves to aggravate PMS symptoms.

ESTROGEN AND SEROTONIN LEVELS

By now, we've strongly established the fact that low levels of serotonin cause depression. The domino effect of the inter-relationship between amino acids, vitamins and neurotransmitters is further complicated by the presence of estrogen. An excess of estrogen can also occur if your hormonal balance is disrupted. An estrogen overload can cause a number of distressing symptoms. Estrogen is a central nervous stimulant while progesterone has the opposite effect. Maintaining the right balance between these two hormones is a complex and delicate process. Any imbalance which may result during PMS, pregnancy or menopause can trigger a change in mood.

In order to have enough serotonin, you need tryptophan, which is necessary for its production. To have enough tryptophan your body must have certain amounts of vitamin B-6. This chemical chain can be broken by estrogen, which can block the action of vitamin B-6 and force it to be eliminated from the body. Estrogen can also speed up the production of tryptophan which, ironically, makes it less likely to form serotonin.

High estrogen levels are usually required for these chemical reactions to occur and most of the time, the presence of estrogen should not be in excess. If you take the pill, however, or are pregnant or about to have your period, estrogen levels can soar, creating a shortage of tryptophan or vitamin B-6. Consequently, you feel like the world is coming to an end. One of the benefits of taking extra vitamin B-6 is that is has been shown to decrease an unfavorable type of estrogen called estradiol in the bloodstream. At the same time, it helps boost progesterone levels, a hormonal shift which is generally considered desirable.

Women who take estrogen to relieve menopausal symptoms may also develop a vitamin B-6 deficiency which may precipitate a depressed mental state. Taking vitamin B-6 if you suffer from PMS is a must. Studies suggest that B-6 may well increase levels of serotonin and dopamine in the brain, two neurotransmitters which are considered to be too low in some women who are plagued with PMS. It's no wonder that so many women feel like they're losing their sanity every month. Wild fluctuations in mood and extreme irritability are common side-effects of PMS. Knowing how estrogen interferes with normal brain biochemistry explains a whole variety of crazed behaviors.

Doctors are slowly catching on to the potential benefits of vitamin B-6. and are beginning to prescribe it in therapeutic doses. Don't wait until its merit is eventually published in medical journals to use it. Louise Tenney, an expert in the field of natural medicine points out that thousands of medical reports published decades ago testify to the undisputed value of nutritional medicine. Tragically, these articles written by qualified medical doctors and scientists do little but gather dust in archival storage rooms. We need to do a lot of unlearning and rediscover the value of therapies long thrown out as being inferior to pharmaceutical drugs. Doctors, in particular, need to re-think and re-evaluate the medicinal role of natural substances like vitamin B-6.

Finally, and thankfully, after decades of denial, PMS is scientifically recognized as a disorder caused by a biochemical imbalance. Interestingly, this particular disruption in body chemistry can also be linked to an increase in monoamine oxidase which breaks down certain neurotransmitters necessary to prevent depression. In light of how fragile hormonal balance is, the fact that almost half of all women between the ages of 30 and 50 suffer from PMS is understandable.

PMS, CARBOHYDRATE, AND CHOCOLATE CRAVINGS

Food cravings, so typical of PMS, can also shed significant light on the relationship between diet, hormones and brain chemistry. In the chapter on carbohydrate cravings and depression, this relationship is explored by Dr. Richard J. Wurtman a professor of neuroscience and specialist in brain chemistry and his wife Judith, a cell biologist and nutritionist. They have uncovered fascinating data on women who suffer from PMS, and why they crave carbohydrates and chocolate in particular.

Research has shown that one of the common denominators in all cases of PMS studied was a magnesium deficiency. Chocolate contains magnesium, however it is also high in caffeine and fat. As mentioned in an earlier chapter, chocolate also contains phenylalanine, an amino acid needed for healthy brain activity. Additional research has also found that women who typically suffer from PMS, strongly crave carbohydrates prior to their periods to make themselves feel better by raising their serotonin levels. Dr. Wurtman suggests that when these women feel this way they eat complex carbohydrates that are low in fats. He suggests, foods like rice, lentils, potatoes, beans, and pasta. Supplementing the diet with vitamin B-6 can also help control the depressive symptoms of PMS. It is believed that increased concentrations of vitamin B-6 can boost the brain's conversion of tryptophan to serotonin, which can result in an elevation of mood.

HOW TO FIGHT MOOD SWINGS ASSOCIATED WITH PMS

Another plus of using vitamin B-6 for PMS is that in combination with magnesium, it can work as an antispasmodic, helping to reduce uterine cramping. Don't forget, along with using the appropriate vitamins and minerals to control the mood altering symptoms of PMS, a change in diet will likely be needed.

Anyone who suffers from PMS should avoid sugar, caffeine, chocolate, tobacco, alcohol, salt, fatty foods, and high fat dairy products. Emphasize whole grains, fresh, raw fruits and vegetables, lean meats and legumes. Supplementing the diet with fiber is also recommended. Reports have shown that vegetarian women, who get adequate B-vitamins have lower blood levels of estradiol, a form of estrogen we can do without.

While PMS may not be totally cured through a nutritional approach, it can be managed. Using therapeutic dosages of magnesium, vitamin B-complex, especially emphasizing vitamin B-6 and vitamin E can help to control some of these troublesome symptoms.

The good news is that several studies have proven that if you supplement your diet with B-6, you have an excellent chance of remaining free from severe depression. If you take birth control pills, be aware that wild fluctuations of blood sugar can also result, causing sugar related depression and other symptoms. Refer to the section of depression and hypoglycemia for more information.

Incidentally, regarding the connection between yeast infections and PMS, Pamela Morford, M.D., a gynecologist in Minneapolis commented: "The premenstrual problems of at least ninety percent of my patients can be traced to chronic candidiasis. I have found that when I give these patients anti-candida therapy, they get better." [93] For more information on the link between mood disorders and candidiasis, see the chapter on yeast infections.

DRUGS THAT CAN CAUSE
DEPRESSION

"Depression is often a side-effect of drug usage,
particularly of substances not often considered drugs,
i.e. oral contraceptives, caffeine and cigarettes."
Michael T. Murray N.D.

If you can't understand why you might feel depressed, before you do anything else, look at any drugs you might be taking. These include both prescription and over-the-counter preparations. Depression can be a side-effect of any drug usage including alcohol, caffeine and nicotine. Anytime we take a drug, we may be disrupting the normal balance of monoamines in the brain which can predict mood.

DRUGS AND GERIATRIC DEPRESSION

An article written in the *Journal of the American Geriatric Society* states: "Drugs, either prescribed by a physician or taken independently, often are responsible for the development of depression, the aggravation of a pre-existing depression or the production of depression-like symptoms such as sedation, apathy and lethargy."[94]

This article goes on to discuss the fact that many elderly people are not suffering from senility but from the depressive side-effects of the myriad drugs they usually consume. It's not uncommon for an older person to take a whole handful of pills, and overdosing routinely occurs.

In addition, new research published in the *Journal of the American Geriatric Society*, reveals that depression, not senility or poor fitting dentures is the real cause of weight loss in most nursing home patients. Depression was found to be the cause of weight loss in 37 percent of 156 nursing home residents who lost five pounds or more.[95] The question here is, how much of that depression was drug-induced? Rarely do geriatric doctors address the issue of the incidence of depression in the elderly, and most geriatric symptoms are shrugged off as part of the aging process.

The first indication that depression might be caused by a biochemical imbalance in the brain came in the 1950's, when several patients who were being treated with resperine for hypertension became depressed. A similar scenario resulted with patients who were given iproniazid, an anti-tuberculosis drug. How many other drugs that we so take so casually cause the same types of mood fluctuations?

STEROIDS AND DEPRESSION

Clearly, using corticosteroids which are commonly prescribed for a host of ailments can cause depression, especially in the young. Physicians in Italy report that one five year old girl given cortisone for chronic hepatitis became increasingly depressed until she was terribly uncommunicative and had uncontrollable crying spells. If you must take steroid drugs, some research has suggested that supplementing the diet with vitamin C may help to counteract this particular side-effect.

OVER-THE-COUNTER AND PRESCRIPTION ANTIHISTAMINES AND MOOD

Certain over-the-counter antihistamine medications can depress the nervous system and make you feel like the world is coming to an end. I've had some experience with this effect during allergy season. I noticed that when I took a 12 hour cold cap, I would feel unusually low, and pessimistic. As long as I took the medication, the depression persisted and my moods continued to drop. The effect was so pronounced that friends and relatives became concerned that my attitude had become so morose.

I don't believe the package referred to this as a possible side-effect, however it most surely was. The small print on the side of the box did mention something about depressing the nervous system. This hardly served as an adequate warning. Anyone who was already suffering from depression and took what they thought were harmless antihistamines, may only compound their problem.

The following list contains other drugs which may cause depression:

SOME ANTIHISTAMINES INCLUDING THOSE CONTAINING
   BENADRYL

ANTIBIOTICS
   Cycloserine (Seromycin)
   Tetraclyclines
   Neomycin
   Metronidazole (Flagyl)
   Sulfonamides (Bactrim, Azo, Gantanol, Cotrim, Septra, Sulfatrim,
      Sulfa Methoxazole)
   Gram Negative Antibiotics
ANTI-INFLAMMATORIES
   Indocin
   Naprosyn
ANTIMALARIALS
   Sulfadoxine
   Pyrimethamine (Daraprim, Fansidar)
ARTHRITIS MEDICATIONS AND PAIN RELIEVERS
   Phenylbutazone (Azolid, Butazolidin)
   Indomethacin (Indocin)
   Piroxicam (Feldene)
   Sulfasalazine (Azulfidine)
   Aspirin (including buffered aspirin)
   Phenacetin (A.P.C. with Codeine, Propoxyphene Compound, Soma
      Compound)
BIRTH CONTROL PILLS AND HORMONES
   Estrogens
   Progesterone
   Steroids

Oral contraceptives can cause several nutrient deficiencies which
are associated with depressive illness. For more information on how to
minimize these effects if you take birth control pills, see the chapter on
Hormones and Depression.

CHEMOTHERAPY
   Vinblastine Sulfate (Velban)
   Methotrexate
   Procarbazine hydrochloride (Matulane)

DIET PILLS
Amphetamines (Obetrol, Dexedrine, Desoxyn)
Benzphetamine (Didrex)
Diethylpropion hydrochloride (Tednuate, Tepanil)
Phenmetrazine hydrochloride (Preludin)
Mazindol (Sanorex Mazanor)
Fenfluramine hydrochloride (Pondimin)
Phendimetrazine tartrate (Plegine, Melfiat, Bontril)
Phentermine (Ionamine, Fastin, Adipex-P)

DIURETICS
Furosemide
Triamterene (Dyazide, Dyrenium)

HEART MEDICATIONS
Digitalis (Digoxin, Lanoxin, Cedilanid, Crystodigin)
Procainamide (Pronestyl, Procan SR)

HIGH BLOOD PRESSURE MEDICATIONS
Hydralazine (Apresazide Apresoline)
Methyldopa (Aldomet, Aldoclor, Aldoril)
Clonidine hydrochloride (Catapres, Combipres)
Guanethidine (Ismelin, Esimil)
Propanolol hydrochloride (Inderal, Inderide)
Bethanidine
Reserpine (Chloroserpine, Regroton, Diupres, Diutensen-R, H-H-R
　　　Tabs, Hydropres, Serpasil, Unipres, Ser-Ap-Es,Naquival,
　　　Metatensin, Hydromox, Hydro-Fluserpine)

PARKINSON'S DISEASE MEDICINE
Amatadine hydrochloride (Symmetrel)
Levodopa (Larodopa, Sinemet)

MEDICATIONS FOR PSYCHOSIS
Phenotiazines (Compazine, Phenergan, Sparine, Stelazine, Temaril,
　　　Thorazine)
Haloperidol (Haldol)
Thioxanthene (Navane)

SEIZURE MEDICATIONS
Succinimide (Celontin, Zarontin, Milontin)
Carbamazepine (Tegretol)
Mephenytoin (Mesantoin)

SLEEPING MEDICATIONS AND TRANQUILIZERS
Librium
Valium
Barbiturates

NOTE: using over-the-counter sleeping aids like Compoz, Ecedrin-P.M., Sleep-Eze3 and Sominex can cause disorientation.

OTHER DRUGS THAT MAY CAUSE DEPRESSION
Disulfiram (Antabuse)
Physostigmine (Antilirium)
Tagamet (can cause nutritional deficiencies if taken for a prolonged
period of time
Choline (in large doses)
Lecithin (contains choline)
Cholestyramine

NICOTINE

If you are suffering from depression, stop smoking. If you're not suffering from depression, stop smoking. Dr. Andrew Weil M.D. tells us that smoking puts drugs into the brain more directly than an intravenous injection.[96] Smoking can affect emotional behavior through the action of carbon monoxide which is toxic to brain cells. In addition, ingesting nicotine can significantly lower vitamin C levels which can lead to depletion symptoms. A lack of vitamin C, as previously discussed, can contribute to a number of neurotic symptoms, including depression.

To make matter worse, smoking stimulates the adrenal glands to secrete adrenaline and cortisol. Cortisol inhibits the uptake of tryptophan by brain cells, which results in lowered levels of serotonin. By now, we should be all too aware that decreased serotonin levels cause depression.

Unknown to most smokers is the fact that nicotine can compound the effect of caffeine and sugar on the system, two more culprits in mood determination. So, if you typically eat a danish for breakfast, and have a cigarette and a coke on your break, you're setting up the perfect biological stage for the development of diseases like depression.

Nicotine belongs to the same family of addictive substances as alcohol, caffeine and sugar. The addiction cycle in each of these is a treacherous one. You feel lousy so you grab a doughnut, you pour yourself a drink, or you light up. The initial result is that you feel better...the long term one is that you'll feel worse. Like any drug, the effects of nicotine are only temporary. Your mood and energy levels will eventually drop, so you start all over again and the destruction goes on.

Smoking is one of the most devastating things you can do to your health. If you want to stop, see your doctor and arm yourself with everything you need to succeed. Determination and the will to stop are going to be your best weapons. Keep in mind that you're going to feel a whole lot worse before you feel better...but you will feel better, 100 percent better.

CAFFEINE:

Caffeine is the most widely used drug in our society. It is found in a number of foods, medications and beverages and the average American consumes 150-225 mg. of caffeine each and every day. We could write a whole chapter on all the negative biological effects of caffeine on the human body. For our purposes, caffeine's effect on brain amines is frightening enough. The intake of caffeine has been positively correlated with the degree of mental illness in psychiatric patients.

People with any kind of mental dysfunction pay a great price for excessively using caffeine. Heavy coffee drinkers score higher on tests for anxiety and depression and are more likely to suffer from psychotic disorders. Caffeine stimulates the release of norepinephrine along with other neurotransmitters in the brain. This explains the immediate lift you experience after you drink a cup of coffee. Consistent overuse of caffeine results in a lack of these same brain amines which affect mood, not to mention its adverse effects on vitamin B-1, iron and magnesium absorption. Remember, a lack of any of these nutrients can contribute to depression.

You need to ingest around 250 milligrams of caffeine to experience mental symptoms. A cup of coffee can contain between 29 to 175 milligrams, a cola beverage 40 milligrams, a chocolate bar, 25 milligrams and several over-the-counter analgesics a varying amount of caffeine. So, if you drink three cups of coffee, take two headache pills, eat a chocolate bar and drink one cola drink, you may have ingested 400 milligrams of caffeine.

Caffeine activates the sympathetic nervous system and can make us feel jittery, anxious or even fearful. Would you reach for your cola big gulp if you knew it contained a mind-altering drug? Well, it does. Caffeine acts a constant annoyance to the nervous system and artificially creates energy. Cocaine and amphetamines work the same way.

Another substance which acts very much like caffeine in the body is phenylpropanolamine (PPA). This chemical is commonly found in over-the-counter diet pills, cold remedies, and decongestants. Be wary of these stimulants. They can actually block your ability to relax and contribute to depressed states of mind. Get rid of them.

ALCOHOL:

Alcohol may well be the most devastating substance in our twentieth century repertoire of drugs and chemicals. Alcoholism is by far our country's number one health problem and the third leading cause of death in the United States. There are twelve million alcoholics in America today, not to mention the additional millions who are considered heavy drinkers. Alcohol has exacted an enormous toll on our society financially, physically and emotionally.

Alcohol can determine mood. It's that simple. One reason that more women than men have drinking problems may be because they struggle more with depression. Consequently, they reach for a drink. The devastating biochemical ramifications of drinking only serves to further compound depression.

Ingesting too much alcohol can create B vitamin, amino acid and mineral deficiencies. You don't have to drink large quantities of alcohol to develop vitamin B depletion. Consistently drinking even small quantities can result in the malabsorption of vitamin B-1, B-2 and folic acid.

To make matters even worse, other nutrients such as vitamin B-6 and C are destroyed by a by-product of alcohol produced in the liver every time you ingest it. Minerals such as zinc, calcium and magnesium are excreted more readily in the urine when alcohol is present in the blood- stream. Some recent studies have suggested that alcohol also decreases the metabolism of certain brain amines formed from tyrosine.

Like any mind-altering drug, it is easy to become dependent on alcohol for your sense of well being or relaxation. If you drink to feel better than you're a prime candidate for addiction. Alcohol will prevent you from confronting your depression. It only serves to potentiate the paralyzing effects of depressive illness.

The writing is on the wall concerning alcohol. Drinking is hazardous to your physical and mental health. If you decide to continue drinking, make sure you supplement your diet with a daily regimen of vitamins and minerals. Vitamin B-1 and B-complex are burned up by alcohol. Much of the nerve damage seen in alcoholics is the result of a thiamine deficiency (vitamin B-1) A much better option is to stop drinking. Get help if you need to.

Undoubtedly, taking drugs of any kind impacts all body systems, not just the targeted ones. The emotional consequences of taking various drugs is seldom discussed by physicians. If you have been taking any of the drugs listed, do not stop unless you have been advised to by your physician. The abrupt withdrawal from a drug can also cause a number of serious problems.

Certain drugs can inhibits the body's vitamin reserves which can not only weaken the immune system, but make the mind vulnerable to depression caused by nutrient depletion. Dr. Daphne, Roe in the October-November, 1973 issue of *Food and Nutrition News* states: "Anticonvulsants, the Pill, and also another pharmacologically unrelated drug, the sedative glutethimide (Doriden), have been found capable of producing multiple vitamin deficiencies." How many other drugs, even seemingly harmless over-the-counter varieties do the same thing?

THE THYROID CONNECTION

"The thyroid gland controls so many aspects of metabolism that distrubance of its function can produce symptoms in almost every system of the body."

Andrew Weil, M.D.

Low thyroid function and depressive illness are intrinsically linked. Because the function of brain amines or neurotransmitters interrelate with the endocrine system, people who are depressed frequently have other hormonal malfunctions. Like the vitamin B deficiency question, it is difficult to assess which comes first: does depression causes the hormonal imbalance or vice versa. A combination of both of these situations is the most probable scenario.

In any case, the hypothalamus is the area in the brain that regulates and balances your body's hormones. Like other brain tissue, it will respond to the chemical environment of the brain, producing the necessary hormones. In order to produce these hormones, you must supply your body with amino acids, essential fatty acids, vitamins, and minerals, which, are ideally derived from a good, nutritious diet. If you're depressed, you most likely suffer from a lack of certain brain chemicals. This deficiency not only makes you feel "blue," it can also initiate hormonal imbalances and metabolic malfunctions. If you have a hormonal imbalance to start with, becoming depressed may be an inevitable outcome of the disorder.

Depression is often the first symptom of thyroid disease. Even a very subtle decrease in thyroid hormone can produce symptoms of depressive illness. Some doctors believe that depression is the major manifestation of a sluggish thyroid gland, referred to as Hypothyroidism. Almost half of all people who suffer from an inactive thyroid also feel depressed.

SYMPTOMS OF AN UNDERACTIVE THYROID GLAND

Typically, anyone who has an underactive thyroid will be chronically tired and unable to get things done at a normal pace. Mornings would be particularly difficult, with a lack of energy being the primary problem. Feeling low or mentally dull can result from this thyroid imbalance. Other symptoms include:
- Excess sleepiness
- Menstrual cycle changes
- Weight gain characterized by swelling and puffy tissues
- Muscle weakness
- Hoarseness
- Constipation
- Lack of perspiration
- Hair loss
- Dry, coarse skin

If you suspect you might have a thyroid problem, see your doctor. Classic symptoms of a hypoactive thyroid are an intolerance to cold and a low basal temperature. Keep in mind that a hypoactive thyroid is not easily diagnosed with designated lab tests. If you have any or a combination of the above symptoms in combination with chronic depression, you should suspect that your thyroid may indeed by sluggish. Pursue this with your doctor, until you are sure you can rule it out. Request T3, T4 and TSH tests. If these are inconclusive, have your doctor run a TRH test as well.

TYROSINE AND THYROID DISORDERS

It is fascinating to learn that in order for the thyroid gland to form its hormone, TSH, tyrosine, an amino acid and iodine are required. It has been proposed that if you have a hypoactive thyroid, your body will channel available tyrosine to the gland to boost the production of thyroid hormone. If this is the case, tyrosine may not be sufficiently available for the production of norepinephrine, a neurotransmitter crucial to maintaining a good mental outlook. As a result, depression will occur.

TREATMENTS FOR HYPOTHYROIDISM

If you suffer from low thyroid, you should see your physician, In addition, you can benefit from supplementing your diet with vitamin B-complex, calcium/magnesium, vitamin C with bioflavonoids, zinc and tyrosine. Stay away from white sugar, white flour, red meats, milk, cheese, eggs and junk foods. Don't smoke, use caffeine or alcohol.

Keep in mind that thyroid medications in correcting hormone levels will usually also relieve the depressive illness. Boosting the amount of thyroid hormone can actually potentiate antidepressive medications, improving their effectiveness. Hopefully, correcting hypothyroidism will eliminate the need for antidepressant drugs all together.

An unorthodox and relatively new treatment designed to stimulate the thyroid gland in people who are depressed is called sleep deprivation. Apparently the periodic controlled absence of sleep can restore normal levels of TSH (thyroid hormone) in some people. See the section in this book on sleep for more details.

Statistics tell us that up to 20 percent of people suffering from depression have a sluggish thyroid. Carefully consider the symptoms of hypothyroidism and insist that you doctor do the necessary tests to either rule out or confirm the disorder. For more information on the connection between the thyroid gland and depression see *Hypothyroidism, The Unsuspected Illness,* by Broda Barnes, M.D.

YEAST INFECTIONS AND DEPRESSION

"Fifty years ago doctors identified Candida Albicans as a frequent cause of vaginal, mouth, throat and gastrointestinal tract infections. Now it's well known to affect almost all body parts, organs, tissues and cells."
John Parks Trowfridge, M.D.

Any woman who has experienced the indescribably misery of a vaginal yeast infection will attest to the fact that its aggravating symptoms can make you feel like your losing your mind. While the burning and itching that accompany yeast infections are exasperating, to put it mildly, there may be a whole lot more going on both physically and mentally.

Dr. Orian Truss, M.D. of Birmingham was one of the first doctors to recognize that mood disorders can be due to the effect of a chronic yeast infection. For over twenty years, he has studied the correlation between yeast infections and a variety of complaints, including depression. His conclusion is that yeast infections, also called candidiasis, affect their victims both physically and psychologically.

Yeast infections are believed to induce a number of mental or neurological disorders. There are several theories which attempt to explain the connection, although at this writing, none are really conclusive. Most experts believe that the presence of candida can disturb the normal balance of intestinal flora which can inadvertently affect mood. One other possibility is that the presence of a yeast infection reduces the ability of the liver to clear the bloodstream of toxic waste.

The fact that candida secretes an identifiable toxin is thought to be the most plausible reason for the myriad of symptoms it can produce in the nervous system. Some of these symptoms include: fatigue, irritability, confusion, mood swings, headaches and depression. This theory is supported by the fact the Dr. K. Iwata, a Japanese scientist claims to have isolated the toxin.

Repeated exposure to a candida overgrowth and resulting toxins is what is believed to cause this "yeast syndrome," which incorporates a number of candida-related disorders. Most medical doctors and scientists are extremely skeptical about the link between yeast infections and depression. Demanding more scientific proof of this relationship usually takes a lifetime to secure, in the meantime, observations like those of Dr. Truss should not be ignored.

As with most new approaches to treating disease, distrust is the rule. Unfortunately, by the time the medical establishment accepts new ideas, they've become old and valuable time has been wasted. Some observant doctors have found that yeast and other fungal infections most commonly accompany depression.

WHAT IS A YEAST INFECTION?

A yeast infection or candidiasis is a generally misunderstood condition. A generalized yeast infection would be a very serious condition and could only occur if the immune system was profoundly weakened. This is not the type of yeast infection that we are referring to. Yeast lives within all of our systems and when the biochemistry of those systems is healthy, the yeast may cause us little problem. Many people experience a sensitivity to yeast that has grown on specific mucous membranes of the body, where the climate is moist and favorable. The vagina and the gastrointestinal tract are both susceptible to yeast infections. A yeast infection occurs when the delicate balance of microorganisms is disrupted. As a result, the yeast can rapidly multiply.

While most of us are exposed to yeast, it becomes a problem for only some of us, especially those of us who are females. The climate of the vagina is perfect for yeast proliferation. Men usually develop the infection somewhere in the digestive system, and in children it can show up in certain diaper rashes, thrush and ear infections.

How do you get a yeast infection? Taking antibiotics can create a favorable environment for this fungus by causing the type of imbalance we've just talked about. Antibiotics not only kill harmful bacteria, they do away with the friendly bacteria we need to maintain the proper ratio of microorganisms. For this reason, if you have to take antibiotics, make sure to take lactobacillus acidophilus to replace lost bacteria.

High blood sugar can also predispose the body to a yeast infection. Yeast infections are commonly seen in people with diabetes. The body changes associated with taking birth control pills and steroids can also affect the internal climate of areas prone to infection. Consuming white sugar, breads that are high in yeast and drinking alcohol can all promote yeast infections in some individuals.

A study of one hundred women in the July, 1984 issue of the *Journal of Reproductive Medicine* found that one's intake of sugar, dairy products and artificial sweeteners had a positive correlation with the incidence of Candida vulvovaginitis. After being placed on a diet which eliminated these substances, more than 90 percent of these women were free from yeast infections for over a year.[97]

Once you've had a yeast infection, you may find that they have a tendency to recur. Once a yeast infection has proliferated, it can create a chemical imbalance in the body that can affect the way amino acids are used. By now, it's pretty clear that amino acids are crucial to preventing and stemming depression.

YEAST INFECTIONS AND MOOD DISORDERS

The body systems that are most affected by a chronic yeast infection are the brain and the female endocrine system. It is the brain connection that we are most interested in. Someone suffering from a chronic yeast infection may have trouble concentrating, may be lethargic, irritable or depressed. The symptoms vary with each person.

A little recognized consequence of yeast infections is that it can make you more sensitive to colds and environmental allergens such as weeds, grasses, or various inhalants. Becoming more and more allergic can result in diverse symptoms of which depression and fatigue are two. Doctors have found that when symptoms of a yeast infection cleared up, sensitivities to food and other potential allergens also improved.

SYMPTOMS OF CANDIDIASIS

THE DIGESTIVE SYSTEM: bloating, cramps, gas, diarrhea and constipation, food intolerance

THE SKIN: eczema, hives, excessive perspiration, acne, psoriasis, nail infections

THE GENITO-URINARY TRACT: FOR WOMEN: PMS including: mood swings, depression, water retention, cramps, craving for sweets, and headaches, vaginal itching and burning, discharge, recurring vaginal or bladder infections, and loss of sexual desire. *FOR MEN:* recurring anal itching, prostatitis, impotence, and genital rashes

THE ENDOCRINE SYSTEM: Thyroid and adrenal glands may be affected.

If you suspect you might suffer from chronic yeast infections, you need to see a doctor. In recent years, it seemed as if every ailment in the book was being attributed to candidiasis. Understandably, these links were quickly scoffed at by most physicians. Despite the lack of credibility that accompanied such claims, physicians are beginning to realize that yeast infections are much more prevalent than previously thought, and that they can result in a myriad of other disorders.

HOW TO TREAT AND PREVENT YEAST INFECTIONS

In order to manage and prevent yeast infections, you need to eliminate white sugar, white flour, quick-cooking grains and yeast breads. Get rid of yeast, mold and fungus foods such as alcoholic beverages, bakery products, aged cheese, vinegar, truffles and caffeine. If you have decided to take Nystatin, which is commonly prescribed by doctors to kill a yeast infection, make sure to take acidophilus to replace the friendly bacteria that is destroyed along with the unfriendly. Taking B-vitamins is unquestionably a good thing to do, however, make sure you get the yeast free kind.

Be aware that while candida may in reality, be over-diagnosed as a catch-all for anything that might ail you, the syndrome exists and is often missed by medical practitioners. A blood test for candidiasis is available from several accredited laboratories and detects the presence of candida antibodies in the bloodstream.

One of the best things you can do to protect yourself against the invasion of candida is to routinely take lactobacillus acidophilus. The friendly bacteria in acidophilus competes with the yeast organisms for bowel wall sites. A daily dose of liquid acidophilus can be an effective "inoculation" for the bowel against the development of this disease.

ENVIRONMENTAL FACTORS AND
DEPRESSION

"Be wary of all the chemicals in your life."
Andrew Weil, M.D.

We live in a world teeming with hidden poisons, toxins and carcinogens. Knowing that in and of itself is depressing. While it may not be a pleasant subject, the effects of certain pollutants, chemicals and metals on the human mind must be addressed.

For example, chronic exposure to certain solvents and heavy metals can produce altered moods and psychological behavior. A number of everyday solvents are also capable of interfering with brain cell biochemistry. Certain paints, varnishes used on furniture and in boat building, and virtually any toxic chemical or fume can be capable of producing a mood disorder. The bottom line is; don't underestimate the negative effects of exposing yourself to toxic substances.

CARBON MONOXIDE

Carbon monoxide which comes from car exhaust, tobacco smoke, and wood burning is a colorless and odorless gas. If you work in a parking garage or have a faulty automobile exhaust system, you may be getting slow doses of this poison. Carbon monoxide robs oxygen from the body including the brain. Brain cells are most sensitive to any kind of oxygen deprivation. As a result, if your brain is oxygen starved, psychiatric symptoms are common. Like so many other conditions that can cause behavioral symptoms, carbon monoxide poisoning can be easily misdiagnosed as schizophrenia or psychotic depression.

INSECTICIDES

Organophosphate insecticides can have the same effect on the nervous system as nerve gas used in chemical warfare. If you are consistently exposed to these chemicals you can become irritable, tense, anxious, restless, depressed and emotionally withdrawn. This family of insecticides inhibit acetylcholinesterase, an essential enzyme in the brain.

OTHER EVERYDAY TOXINS AND POLLUTANTS

People who work with paints, varnishes, refinery workers, people who manufacture or use pesticides, and people who routinely handle fuel may be at risk for developing personality changes, panic disorders, irritability and depression.

Engaging in potentially lethal habits like sniffing glue, gasoline, cleaning fluid and nitrous oxide can also create mental disorders. The initial euphoria that results from these kinds of activities turns into conduct-disordered behavior. Exposure to these kind of chemicals creates abnormal behavior which can be misinterpreted as a psychiatric disorder.

The connection between exposure to heavy metals and depression is well documented. Of the naturally occurring elements, 69 are metals. Today, our usage of metals has become more clever and sophisticated. Metals are found in fuels, medicines, makeup, hair spray, kitchen cleaners, herbicides and insecticides.

The recent link between aluminum salts and Alzheimer's disease has not been scientifically resolved yet its possibility looms. We routinely ingest aluminum in salt, some antacids, and cake mixes, just to name a few sources. Ingesting or breathing lead, mercury or radioactive metals can wreak havoc with the human body and create psychiatric mayhem with the human mind. The brain is more sensitive to these metals than other parts of the body, therefore, mental and behavioral symptoms may be more obvious than physical signs of poisoning.

Too much or too little magnesium, calcium, zinc, lead, mercury, bismuth, aluminum, bromides, lithium, thallium and organophosphates can cause clinical depression.

If you overuse diuretics you can develop a sodium or potassium deficiency serious enough to cause harmful physical and mental symptoms. A lack of iron can make you feel depressed and irritable and too much iron can be life-threatening. If you have a thyroid disorder or pancreatitis, you can develop serious symptoms of a calcium overload in the blood which can manifest itself as depression or psychiatric illness.

A condition referred to as manganese madness can occur in people who work in manganese mines or steel foundries where manganese dust is inhaled. In these cases, depression is typical.

One very good reason for taking vitamin and mineral supplements in dosages higher than the RDA is to protect our bodies against the rampant and often hidden environmental toxins we encounter each and every day. We've all heard the term "free radicals" which refers to molecules which are extremely reactive because they contain an unpaired electron. Free radicals cause damage to the human body. Common sources of free radicals are car exhaust, herbicides, pesticides, drugs, cigarette smoke, radiation, food additives, industrial waste, and polluted air.

PROTECTING YOURSELF AGAINST SUBSTANCES THAT ALTER BRAIN CHEMISTRY

If you regularly take antioxidant nutrients such as vitamin C with bioflavonoids, you can help neutralize the devastating biological effects of free radicals. Keep in mind that the RDA requirement for vitamin C does not take the factor of toxin exposure into account when it determines its quotas. In reality, most of us eat lousy diets, many of us smoke and drink alcohol and all of us are subject to stress and toxin exposure. Perhaps, if we lived in a utopic society, the RDA requirements would suffice. The truth is that we don't.

If you are suffering from unexplained depression, examine your home and work environment and make sure you're not continually exposed to harmful toxins without protection. Take plenty of vitamin C with bioflavonoids along with other nutritive supplements. Your sanity may depend on it.

DEPRESSION AND HERBS

"Herbs and plants are medical jewels gracing the woods, fields, and lanes, which few eyes see, and few minds understand. Through this want of observation and knowledge the world suffers immense loss"

Linnaeus

After founding the Bio-Brain Center in Princeton, N.J., Dr. Karl Pfeiffer stated, "For every drug that benefits a patient, there is a natural substance that can achieve the same effect."

It has been estimated that as much as 75 percent of the population of this planet relies on herbal medicine. What is not commonly known is that this widespread use of herbs is not limited to poor or backward nations. Almost half of all medical doctors in France and Germany use herbal therapy as part of their healing strategies. For some reason, this isn't the case in our country. Herbs have gained an unsavory reputation, (no pun intended), and in so doing, have been cast aside by most members of the medical community as archaic and superstitious treatments. The assumption that there is no scientific evidence to support the therapeutic use of herbs is not accurate. Scientific research on plants and their use as medicinal agents has been mounting over the last few years.

Over the last two decades, there has been a large proliferation of scientific data regarding herbal therapies. The findings show that for many disorders, herbs provide safer and even more effective treatments than do some prescription drugs. Generaly speaking, herbs are much less toxic than drugs, consequently, they have far less side-effects. Differentiating between the way herbs work versus drugs is crucial to understanding their healing value. The mechanics of many herbs function in the body to correct the cause of a specific illness, while synthetic drugs are geared toward alleviating symptoms of illness.

Using herbs to treat disease is part of the holistic approach toward getting well, which addresses the needs of the mind and spirit as well as the body. Recently, much has been published regarding the body/mind connection. It would be wise to assume that total health depends on the harmonious integration of the physical, the emotional, and the spiritual. In light of the nature of depressive illness, this philosophy would be particularly valuable. Using herbs is compatible with the overall message of this book, which is to become sufficiently in-tune with our own bodies that we can recognize disease symptoms as they develop and seek out the appropriate treatment. No doubt, herbs, like any other healing agents should not be viewed as cure alls. Botanicals can, however, provide significant relief for a number of depression related ailments which inevitably results in a much better quality of life.

As mentioned earlier, using herbs to treat disease usually raises a few eyebrows among conventional health care providers. Undeniably, the misuse of herbology can be an invitation to reckless quackery. By the same token, the deletion of herbal medicines from treatment itineraries constitutes a gross oversight. Herbs, used properly can help to gently treat hundreds of disease and usually do not have the negative side-effects of most powerful pharmaceutical preparations.

From times of antiquity, herbs have played a profound role in the oral and written healing systems of every culture. Recently, an unprecedented interest has developed concerning herbs and their medicinal value. If mainstream medicine is going to accept herbal therapies as valid treatment options, good, reliable scientific data and chemical analysis regarding herbs must become available. In the meantime, herbalism, whether it is scientifically supported or based on empirical data should not be dismissed.

Herbs can be taken in dried form, usually available in capsules, or as teas, extracts or tinctures. The benefits of aromatic chemicals that come from essential oils for mood disorders has been taught for centuries. These aromas are believed to reach brain centers responsible for emotion and either have a stimulating or sedating effect. It's no wonder that smells have the power to evoke strong emotional responses based on past experiences. Aromatic herbs can affect our emotions and mood.

ANCIENT VIEWS OF DEPRESSSION

Depression in ancient medicine was traditionally linked with a disruption of the "melancholic" humor in Galenical medicine. The Chinese have viewed depression as a disturbance in the chi or natural energy of the human body and would recommend chi-moving herbs to treat mood disorders. Regarding mood disorders, the crown chakra which is associated with the pineal gland would be targeted for treatment with herbs like gotu kola and nutmeg.

In the terms of Ayurveda, which is derived from two Indian words: ayur or life, and veda or knowledge, depression is seen as a disruption of the state of vata and kapha which directly effects the nerves. Eastern medicine considers any emotional disorder as a possible cause of a number of diseases, and herbs are routinely used to treat depressive illness. Invariably, all ancient practices view the body as part of an integrated whole. In light of this approach, depression like other diseases is considered a disruption in the ideal balance of body systems which creates health.

While all of this may sound a bit like hocus pocus, there is much to be gleaned from centuries of herbal medicine. If you carefully interpret what may sound like bizarre views in comparison to modern day clinical explanations, you often find a sound scientific basis for ancient perceptions.

Depression can be a disruption of a delicate biochemical balance that is affected by a number of body systems. If one gets out of whack, in domino fashion, several others are thrown off. The insidious sugar cycle is a good example. You crave sugar because you are nutritionally deficient which, in itself creates a deficit of certain brain amines that produce feelings of vigor and well being. You eat sugar which makes you feel better at first, but eventually disrupts hormonal balances, blood sugar levels and even vitamin B assimilation. Inevitably, you become mentally and physically exhausted again, so you reach for a candy bar and the loop goes on.

HOW TO USE HERBAL TREATMENTS

Herbal therapies have the capability of to help control depression by augmenting all body systems. Because herbs are considered foods as well as natural medicines, they also supply the body with vitamins and minerals. The fact that herbs are sometimes classified as food does not imply that they can be randomly ingested. While herbs usually do not have the toxicity or side-effects of pharmaceutical drugs, they must be used with caution and in recommended dosages. Herbs, like any medicine should be gradually tapered on to and off of. Keep in mind also that just because something is considered an herb, it is not necessarily good for depression. Guarana contains large amounts of caffeine and should be avoided all together.

In designing an herbal regimen for the treatment of depression four body systems must be considered: 1.) the endocrine system, which controls hormonal secretions such as insulin and brain biochemistry, 2.) the nervous system, which can influence mood and mental state, 3.) the liver, which can help detoxify excess estrogen and other toxic substances, and 4.) the intestinal system, which must function properly to eliminate waste and toxins from the body.

In addition, specific symptoms which accompany depression can also be treated individually with specific herbs. For example, fatigue can be treated with a number of energy promoting herbs which have been used for centuries to reinvigorate the nervous system and boost stamina and endurance. In addition, several herbs which have been traditionally used for elevating mood are also listed.

In choosing herbal remedies, you must carefully evaluate your state of health. If you know you are hypoglycemic, or suffer from chronic yeast infections etc., select herbs that will specifically treat those disorders. If insomnia is a problem, there are a variety of herbs which are wonderful substitutes for potentially harmful hypnotic drugs. Taking herbal preparations to induce sleep is far superior to becoming addicted to strong prescription drugs like Valium.

The herbs which have been included in this book have been chosen on the basis of their merit and track record. If you choose to try any of them, consult a qualified health practitioner to help you decide on proper dosages. Don't stop any medications you may be taking in favor of herbal therapies. If you want to stop taking a particular drug, discuss this with your doctor and proceed only with his approval and supervision.

A discussion on Aromatherapy will follow with a subsequent listing of specific herbs chosen for their ability to treat symptoms of depression.

MEDICINAL HERBS FOR TREATING INDIVIDUAL SYMPTOMS ASSOCIATED WITH DEPRESSION

NOTE: Anytime you use herbs, you must make sure that you purchase pure herbal products and that you use them judiciously. Herbs, unlike drugs, rarely produce overnight results and must be taken consistently over an extended period of time.

CAUTION: Never stop taking an antidepressant or any other drug without the supervision of your doctor. Mixing certain herbs and drugs can also be undesirable and should only be done under your doctor's care.

HERBS TO INCREASE ENERGY AND COMBAT MENTAL FATIGUE:

GOTU KOLA (Hydrocotyle asiatica)
Parts used: plant

Gotu Kola has traditionally been used to treat the mental and physical fatigue that so commonly accompany depression. It has employed as a botanical medicine since prehistoric times in both India and Indonesia. Gotu Kola is considered a natural nervous system stimulant and helps the body dispose of excess fluid, acting as a natural diuretic.

Gotu Kola has been referred to as an herbal brain food that can help rebuild energy reserves and promote stamina. It has been utilized in the treatment of schizophrenia, epilepsy and memory loss. If you are pregnant or nursing, or have any gastrointestinal disorders, you should avoid taking this herb. Gotu Kola contains vitamins A and K and is rich in magnesium

GINSENG (Panex spp)
Parts used: root

Ginseng is a widely used Oriental herb which can help combat stress and fatigue. It has been used in China for over 5000 years and is undoubtedly the most famous Chinese medicinal plant. Scientific studies have shown that Ginseng has the ability to revitalize both the physical and mental systems of the body. Double blind studies have supported the fact that Ginseng does indeed enhance well being and performance. Practically speaking, Ginseng is a particularly good herb for anyone suffering from weakness, lethargy or a lack of energy. Its anti-fatigue properties are useful for anyone suffering from depressive illness.

In addition, Ginseng is considered a glandular tonic. It stimulates brain and heart function and can decrease blood sugar levels. Ginseng has also been taken to increase mental alertness and overcome lethargy. Ginseng contains vitamins A, B-12 and E.

GINKGO (Ginkgo biloba)
Parts used: leaves and seeds

Ginkgo has been recently re-discovered for its mental and physical benefits. In 1985, Rudolf Weiss stated regarding Ginkgo therapy: "Significant improvement in mental states, emotional lability, and tendency to tire easily have been reported..."

Ginkgo seems to have the ability to boost blood supply to the brain, which results in improved mental functions including memory. Because more blood gets to the brain, glucose, its main energy source is utilized more efficiently. In a French double-blind study of 166 patients with cerebral disorders, treatment with Ginkgo resulted in improved mental alertness, mobility, communication and orientation.[99]

Ginkgo is well suited for long term use and appears extremely safe if taken in prescribed dosages. It is especially good for stress and mental fatigue. It is considered an adaptogen herb which helps the body deal with any kind of stressful situation.

The most effective Ginkgo contains 24 percent ginkgo flavoglycosides. Currently, there is a glut of Ginkgo on the market. Make sure to check your sources for potency and quality. Ginkgo is considered safe enough to use for an extended period of time.

MARJORAM, MINT, VERBENA AND THYME

These herbs are classified as energizing herbs which can be used to replace caffeine. Making teas out of these herbs is believed to help invigorate the body and mind. Using Marjoram and Thyme oil is also recommended as aromatherapy for melancholia. Use the oil in fragrance simmer pots or put it directly on a cotton ball where its fragrance will be easily detected. Flowering Lemon and Orange oil can have the same effect.

CAYENNE (Capsicum frutescens)
Parts used: fruit

Cayenne or Capsicum helps to stimulate circulation and has an energizing effect on the system. It has traditionally been used for overcoming fatigue and restoring stamina and vigor. It is considered a natural stimulant without the side-effects of most stimulating agents. It is high in vitamins A, C, iron and calcium.

HERBS TO HELP REGULATE AND BALANCE HORMONES

DONG QUAI (Angelica Sinensis)
Part used: root

The reputation of this herb in the Orient is second only to Ginseng. This particular herb is useful in achieving hormonal balance and can be used to help with depression that is associated with female problems. Recent studies have proven the ability of Dong Quai to help achieve estrogen equilibrium.

Dong Quai has been used for thousands of years in the Orient to help remedy female disorders caused by hormonal imbalances and is referred to as a tonic for the female glandular system. It is also believed to tranquilize the central nervous system. Dong Quai is naturally rich in vitamin E, B-12, cobalt and iron. It is considered a tonic for the female endocrine system and a natural rejuvenator.

If taken in recommended dosage, long term use of Dong Quai is appropriate.

BORAGE (Borago officinalis)
Part used:leaves

John Gerard, an renown herbalist, used this particular quote: ego borago gaudia semper ago, which means, "I Borage always bring courage." Modern medical research has found that Borage stimulates the adrenal glands, which results in increased energy and initiative. Borage is considered a restorative for the adrenal cortex and is also believed to help ease depression.

CHASTE TREE (Vitex agnuscastus)
Part used: berries

This herb acts on the pituitary gland to help stimulate and normalize hormone function. It works well when combined with vitamin B supplements.

BLACK COHOSH (Cimicifuga racemosa)
Parts used: rhizome

Black Cohosh has been used medicinally by Native Americans who harvested it in forests found in the Eastern United States and Canada. Black Cohosh is a traditional remedy for the mental and emotional disturbances that usually accompany PMS and childbirth. It helps to regulate hormones and exerts a calming influence on the central nervous system. It also provides calcium and magnesium, which are considered nervines. Black Cohosh should not be taken in large amounts and should be purchased from a reliable source

HERBS TO CALM AND STABILIZE THE NERVES AND TO PREVENT INSOMNIA

CHAMOMILE (Anthemis nobilis)
Parts used: flower

This herb has been used for generations to help pacify and soothe raw nerves. A cup of Chamomile tea taken prior to bed has been a traditional favorite for generations for its ability to promote sleep and calm the nervous system. This particular herb is commonly used in France and Spain for its safe, sedating effect. Chamomile also contains significant amounts of calcium, magnesium, zinc, manganese and iron.

PASQUE FLOWER (Anemone pulsatilla)
Part used: aerial portions

Pasque flower is considered a nervine herb and has natural sedative action. It is used to help ease nervous tension and excessive stress. It can be combined with Jamaican Dogwood if anxiety is extreme. It should be used in dried form only.

SKULLCAP (Scutellaria lateriflora)
Parts used: roots and aerial portions

This herb was traditionally used by Native Americans long before Europeans discovered its medicinal properties. Today, it is considered one of the best herbs for treating nervous disorders. David Hoffman, in *The Holistic Herbal* refers to Skullcap as "the most widely relevant nervine available to us in the materia media." Skullcap is an herbal relaxant and restorative for the central nervous system. It is traditionally used as a tonic for any kind of nervous prostration. When combined with wood betony, lavender and lemon balm, its calming effect is enhanced.

WOOD BETONY (Stachys officinalis)
Parts used: aerial and root portions

Wood Betony is thought to be the most important of all Anglo-Saxon herbs. A Saxon translation from the Herbarium Apuleii relates that "it is good whether for a man's soul or his body."

This herb is used to help promote a feeling of emotional stability and is also good for anxiety or irritability.

VERVAIN (Verbena officinalis)
Parts used: aerial portions

This herb was one of the Druid's most venerated medicinal plants. It was referred to as the sacred plant by the Romans, who used it to purify their temples of undesirable influences. Vervain is a traditional, relaxing herbal nervine and tonic that can be combined with Chamomile. Using Vervain tea is recommended for insomnia or other nervous afflictions.

VALERIAN ROOT (Valeriana officinalis)
Parts used: root

Valerian Root is used to calm and stabilize the autonomic nervous system and has been used in Germany to treat depression, PMS, anxiety and postmenopausal symptoms. It has been widely used in folk medicine as a natural sedative. Recent studies have supported the ability of Valerian Root to improve sleep quality and relieve insomnia.[100] These studies also showed that not only was sleep significantly improved with valerian, but the typical hangover associated with prescription hypnotic drugs was not a side-effect. Ironically, Valarian was found to actually decrease morning grogginess.

Clinical studies have shown that Valerian Root preparations appear to stabilize the autonomic nervous system in psychosomatic patients and those with other disorders of the autonomic nervous system. Valerian Root is also believed to promote increased physical and mental performance while it acts as a moderate sedative. It does not have any of the hypnotic or depressive side-effects of tranquilizing drugs. If the herb is used as a tranquilizer, it does not promote sluggishness or lethargy.

German studies have found Valerian Root to be particularly helpful in relieving symptoms of restlessness and stress. It is considered a safe, non-narcotic herbal sedative and is used for anxiety and insomnia. It is not recommended for prolonged use.

PASSION FLOWER: (Passiflora incarnata)
Parts used: leaves

This herb is also considered a natural hypnotic and has been used in Italy to treat hyperactive children. Considered a quieting and soothing nervine, Passion Flower is ideal for anyone who wishes to discontinue using sleeping pills or tranquilizers. This particular herb does not cause depression or disorientation in exchange for its sleep promoting properties.

LAVENDER (Lavandula spp.)
Parts used: flower

Lavender is unquestionably one of the most popular botanicals used since antiquity. It is a natural relaxant and is useful for treating nervous exhaustion. It has been traditionally used to help alleviate mental strain. It can be taken as a tea or put into a sachet that can be placed close to your pillow. Putting Lavender into a warm bath taken one hour before you go to bed can help to relax the body and promote sleep.

HERBS TO HELP ELEVATE MOOD

OATS (Avena sativa)
Parts used: oatstraw and grain

Oats is considered an antidepressant and restorative nerve tonic. It is considered an energy stimulant and is a staple herb in the countries of No. Europe. If your are sensitive to gluten, use Oats only as a clear liquid, which is obtained after the tincture is allowed to settle. Oatstraw is not only considered good for depressive illness, it can also be useful in treating thyroid and estrogen deficiencies, which can result in mood disorders.

ST. JOHN'S WORT (Hypericum perforatum)
Parts used: flowering tops and aerial portions

St. John's Wort has been used for generations as a natural mood elevator. It has the traditional reputation of lightening the mood and lifting the spirits. During the middle ages, it was believed to cast out evil spirits and was consequently used to treat the insane. Recent research has discovered that certain components contained in this herb such as hypericin do indeed alter brain chemistry. It is this biochemical effect on the brain that promotes the improvement of mental outlook.

Clinical studies have shown that St. John's Wort is not only useful for treating depression but can help alleviate anxiety and feelings of worthlessness as well.[101] These studies went as far as to suggest that this herb in extract form may actually be more effective that amitriptyline (Elavil) and imipramine (Tofranil). The side-effects of these two drugs are substantial as discussed in an earlier chapter. By contrast, St. John's Wort has no significant side-effects. This herb can be taken as a tea, an extract or in capsulized form.

One clinical study of 15 depressed women showed that using an extract of St. John's Wort resulted in significant improvement. Symptoms including anxiety and feelings of worthlessness were alleviated with the therapeutic use of this herb. The extract also seemed to have an unexpected bonus, which was to improve the quality of sleep. It proved to be a valuable treatment for the insomnia that frequently accompanied depression.[102]

BASIL (Ocimum basilicum)
Parts used: leaves

Basil has been looked to for generations for its ability to provide a spiritual and emotional lift. It was used extensively during the Middle Ages for melancholia and depression. It is considered an herbal antidepressant and has been found to be particularly effective as a mood elevating aroma. One way to use Basil for depression is to combine Geranium or Rose Oil to Basil Oil and use it in conjunction with massage therapy designed to stimulate. This particular use of Basil is believed to be of significant value in the treatment of depression. Adding Basil Oil to bath water can be an invigorating experience. Basil can also be eaten fresh or taken in capsule form.

Using Basil Oil for aromatherapy is highly recommended for depression. Basil and Neroli, like Marjoram and Thyme are fragrances which fight melancholia and naturally elevate mood. Combining Soy Oil, two drops of Marjoram and 2 drops of Basil Oil creates a wonderful rubbing oil that can ease tension and invigorate.

PEPPERMINT (mentha spp)
Parts used: aerial portions

Peppermint has a long history of use for invigorating the mind and improving the mood. It has been used in tea or oil form to relax tension, ease anxiety and promote of feeling of well being. Its use with message therapy may also prove beneficial for its ability to elevate mood.

DAMIANA (Tunera diffusa)

Parts used: aerial portions

This herb stimulates the nervous system and is called a natural antidepressant. It works well with Oats as a nerve tonic.
An added plus of Damiana for women is its ability to help achieve hormonal balance. It is considered beneficial for both mental and physical exhaustion.

NEROLI OIL (C. aurantium)

Neroli Oil is extracted from Orange blossoms and is an essential oil that is considered particularly effective in combating melancholia and anxiety. Combining 3 drops of this oil with 2 drops of Soy of Almond Oil and then rubbing into the temples, nape of the neck and shoulders can produce an immediate feeling of relaxation. Putting a few drops of Neroli Oil into a warm bath before retiring can promote sleep and prevent insomnia.

EVENING PRIMROSE OIL (Oenothera biennis)
Parts used: seed and oil

This oil is believed to help control mood swings that are characterized by anxiety, and irritability. It contains GLA (gamma-linolenic acid) which is important for glandular health and proper hormonal regulation. It is also high in potassium and magnesium.

LADY'S SLIPPER (Cypripedium pubescens)
Parts used: root

Lady's Slipper acts as a tonic for the central nervous system and helps to calm the emotions. It is considered the safest and most effective nervine botanical in the plant world.

HERBS THAT STIMULATE THE APPETITE:

NUTMEG (myristica fragrans)
Parts used: kernel

First brought to Europe by the Portuguese in 1512, nutmeg became a popular cure-all tonic. It is considered a natural appetite stimulant and when applied externally as an essential oil, can help promote a feeling of well being and energy. Nutmeg is also good for digestive ailments such a nausea and indigestion.

GENTIAN (Gentiana lutea)
Parts used: root

Gentian can help wake up the appetite. Like Nutmeg, it is considered a stomach tonic and has been used to help weak or debilitated patients regain their strength. It also helps to boost sluggish digestion. Gentian is rich in iron and contains B-complex vitamins.

HERBS THAT FIGHT YEAST INFECTIONS

GARLIC (Allium sativum)
Parts used: cloves

For over 5000 years Garlic has been used as a natural antibiotic and immune system stimulant. If you suffer from recurring yeast infections, you should take it on a regular basis. Garlic is available in odorless capsules and can be quite effective in fighting bacterial, fungal and viral infections.

Several recent studies have shown Garlic to have antimicrobial activity against many bacteria, viruses, worms and fungi.[103] Its effectiveness against Candida albicans (yeast infection) has been rated better than nystatin, gentian violet and other antifungal agents.

Garlic helps boost the functions of the immune system and can help prevent the onset of a yeast infection if taken regularly. Hippocrates advised the eating of Garlic as a treatment for cancerous tumors. An additional plus of Garlic is that it helps to lower blood cholesterol and may reduce high blood pressure. Garlic is also a natural source of vitamin A, C and B-1. Garlic can be taken in capules that have been "deodorized."

PAU D'ARCO (Tabebuia avellanedae)

Parts used: inner bark

Pau d'Arco tea contains several properties that fight infection and fortify the immune system. Drinking Pau d'Arco tea is especially recommended. In addition to fighting fungal infections, this herb is rich in calcium and iron. Pau d'Arco is a strong herb but exhibits no harmful side effects. Care must be exercised when purchasing this herb. Many third world sources are heavily contaminated with pesticides. Request only organically wood-grown plants.

POT MARIGOLD (Calendula officinalis)
Parts used:petals

The gold flowers of the marigold plant have been a traditional favorite with herbalists. Pot Marigold is considered an antifungal herb that can be used internally or externally for Yeast infections.

HERBS THAT HELP TO CONTROL HYPOGLYCEMIA

LICORICE (Glycyrrhiza glabra)
Part used: root

Used since 500 B.C. Licorice has been called the grandfather of all herbs. It helps to strengthen the adrenal glands and is believed to boost the effectiveness of glucocorticoids found in the liver. Licorice has been one of the most extensively investigated botanical medicines. It is also believed to help the body cope with stress and to promote a feeling of well being. Some herbalists also use Licorice as an estrogen stimulant. Licorice can also help to balance estrogen levels which can be linked with sugar metabolism. Licorice contains vitamins E, B-complex, biotin, niacin and pantothenic acid. Make sure to take Licorice in recommended dosages. An excess of this herb can cause potassium to be lost and sodium to be retained. If you have a history of hypertension, kidney disease or take heart medications, it's best not to take Licorice.

DANDELION (Taraxacum offinale)

Parts used: leaves and roots

Dandelion has been used as a natural liver tonic for decades and is believed to help regulate blood sugar levels by boosting liver function where glucocorticoids are stored. Dandelion is also a natural source of protein and is rich in vitamin A. It also contains significant amounts of Vitamins B, E, and C and potassium and iron.

GOLDEN SEAL (Hydrastis canadensis)
Part used: rhizome and root

The Cherokee and Iroquois tribes used Golden Seal for a variety of ailments. Golden Seal is a versatile herb that helps to normalize blood sugar levels and has been used for adult onset diabetes. It helps to boost sluggish glands and normalize liver functions which directly impact blood sugar levels. If you take Golden Seal and your blood sugar drops too low, substitute Myrrh instead.

HERBS THAT WORK TO NORMALIZE THYROID FUNCTION

KELP (Fucus versiculosus)
Parts used: whole plant

Kelp grows naturally on Pacific ocean coastlines and is rich in trace minerals. Kelp is also an excellent source of natural iodine which is essential to the proper functioning of the thyroid gland. As a result, it has secondary benefits for the pituitary, adrenal, pineal and parathyroid glands as well. Kelp is believed by some experts to expedite metabolic processes. It has so many beneficial effects on a number of body systems it has been referred to as a systems "sustainer." Kelp contains over 25 minerals and is rich calcium, and B-vitamins as well as iodine.

HERBS THAT PROMOTE GOOD COLON

HEALTH AND ELIMINATION

CASCARA SAGRADA (Rhamnus purshiana)
Parts used: bark

This herb is derived from a tree bark which increases the peristalsis of the colon and has been used for generations to treat constipation. Cascara Sagrada is considered one of the most effective herbal treatments of chronic constipation because it is not habit forming. In addition, this herb is believed to function as a tonic for the nerves and contains B vitamins, calcium, potassium and manganese.

SENNA (Cassia senna)
Parts used: leaves

This herb is considered a good natural laxative because it helps to move waste material through the large intestine by stimulating the action of the colon. If taken with Ginger or Fennel, cramping, which sometimes results as a side-effect can be minimized.

BURDOCK (Arctium lappa)
Parts used: root

Burdock is a traditional cleansing and blood purifying herb. Burdock is a root plant and helps to loosen hard material from the bowel which can impair nutrient absorption. In addition, it assists the pituitary gland in achieving hormonal balance. It also contains a substantial amount of vitamin C and iron.

BARBERRY (Berberis vulgaris)
Parts used: bark

A natural cleanser for the colon, Barberry helps to facilitate the movement of waste material through the colon. Barberry is also considered a liver stimulant which affects other body systems. Barberry is high in vitamin C and contains iron, manganese and phosphorus.

PSYLLIUM (Plantago ovata)

Parts used: seeds

Psyllium seeds function as a bulking laxative for a sluggish or irritable bowel. For this reason, Psyllium is commonly used as an intestinal cleanser. It is ideal because it does not usually irritate the mucous membranes of the intestines. Psyllium is an excellent source of fiber and is frequently found in over-the-counter laxative preparations.

HERBS TO HELP YOU STOP SMOKING

LOBELIA (Lobelia inflata)
Parts used: leaves

Lobelia or Indian tobacco as it is also known contains lobeline. This particular chemical has some of the same effects as nicotine but is not to be confused with nicotine. It has been used orally to inhibit the urge to smoke. Lobelia is a strong herb that must be taken in prescribed dosages. Check with a doctor who is willing to help you try Lobelia. Lobelia also contains sulphur, iron, cobalt, selenium, sodium, and copper.

AROMATHERAPY

"An unexpected whiff of a familiar but long forgotten scent can precipitate a rush of emotions fraught with nostalgia, delirious joy or unspeakable sorrow with more impact than any other form of recollection."

Anonymous

Aromatherapy has been around for centuries. Fragrant oils were used by the ancient Egyptians and Israelites, not to mention a number of Eastern cultures. Dr. Rene-Maurice Gattefosse, who is considered the father of modern aromatherapy has stated: "doctors and chemists will be surprised at the wide range of odoriferous substances which may be used medicinally."

Aromatic oils are commonly used in foods, perfumes, and medicines. Essential oils are concentrated aromatics that will easily evaporate when exposed to air. They are extracted from fragrant plants and are partially soluble in water. Because heat, light and moisture compromise the integrity of these oils, they are kept in dark, air tight bottles.

Various studies conducted to assess the psychological effects of essential oils conclude they can either stimulate or calm the nervous system. At the University of Milan, depressed patients were treated using a combination of Sandalwood, Orange, Verbena, Lemon and Jasmine Oils. For anxiety, Bergamot, Neroli, Cypress, Orange Leaf, Lime and Marjoram were applied.

Doctors at the University of Milan clinically demonstrated the benefit of certain aromatic essences in relieving states of anxiety and depression.[98] The citrus oils they derived from plants were indigenous to Italy...Bergamot, Lemon, and Orange, and were found to successfully elevate mood and dissipate depressive illness. Patchouli Oil has been employed for a number of years in European mental institutions to prevent psychotic reactions and Bergamot is what is traditionally used to treat manic depression.

The validity of aromatherpay has spawned considerable controversy in conventional medical circles. It's therapeutic mechanics involve using natural oils from botanicals rather than chemical agents to initiate a desired effect on the limbic system. Most of us are aware of the bad reputation that "sniffing something" has received over the past few years. By the same token, if inhaling caustic substances can produce bad neurological symptoms, then the opposite must also be true.

According to Dr. Claudia S. Miller M.D. M.S., there are three physical routes through both the nose and the mouth in which substances can affect, stimulate or even cross over into brain tissue. The limbic system of the brain is where mood, short-term memory, long-term memory and smells are stored and interrelate.

Specific smells in the limbic system act as stimuli, consequently, certain neurotransmitters are released. Here we go again. Some smells, particularly chemical oils can produce extremely unpleasant emotional reactions. Whereas, natural oils can evoke a variety of pleasant sensations, not to mention the elevation of mood.

The use of herbals in the form of essentials oils for their aromatic therapeutic value can also greatly benefit anyone who is depressed. Using these oils in combination with face, back, leg and foot massage, putting them in baths, facial saunas, and steamers, and making compresses and poultices with them are the best ways to make the most of their medicinal value. An unusual way to use fragrant oils is to place the drops on a brown sugar cube. A combination of Chamomile, Jasmine, and Bergamot is recommended for depression. Other essences that are considered mood elevators include: Lavender, Clarly Sage, Melissa, and Tiferet-Lifetree.

Specific herbal essential oils have been chosen as possible therapeutic agents in this chapter. How to use them is discussed in conjunction with their description.

For more information on Aromatherapy see:

***Aromatherapy The Complete Guide to Plant and Flower Essences for Health and Beauty* by Danielle Ryman**

MEDITATION, BREATHING, RELAXATION AND SLEEP:
The Ultimate Emotional Elixir

"Contemplate thy powers, contemplate thy wants and thy connections; so shalt thou discover the duties of life, and be directed in all thy ways."

Akhenaton

By now, we've established the fact that if you're suffering from depressive illness you probably need to alter your brain biochemistry to get well. This particular healing approach, however, is not a cure-all for low moods. If you do not learn to re-program your thought patterns and eliminate negative mind-sets, all the biochemistry in the world may ultimately prove useless.

STRESSORS AND MOOD

The little voice that goes with us everywhere and continually provides us with an hour to hour analysis of who we are and how we fit can either make us or break us. If you choose to focus on despair, suffering, injustice and tragedy, you will see it in such overwhelming proportions that nothing else will be visible. Dealing with everyday stressors is an excellent example of how negative factors can overtake our ability to feel happy or well.

Today, the market for any sort of stress reliever is tremendous. Stress reduction has become a multi-million dollar industry. Obviously, most of us feel overly stressed from time to time. Some of us may become depressed because we find we can't adequately cope with our particular kind of stress, or we just find the whole darn business of life overwhelming in itself.

Asking someone who might be depressed if they are dealing with any unusually high stressors is a rather naive question. Who isn't dealing with significant stress in their lives? The cold hard fact is that we cannot eradicate stress from our lives. It is an inherent part of our world. Instead of trying to eliminate all stress, which is usually nothing more than an exercise in futility, we should learn to manage it. Hans Selye views stress as a positive thing. He states, " Stress is the spice of life. Complete freedom from stress is death." Having troubles is the great common denominator which all of us share. It can bind us together as we all struggle to conquer those monsters which would crush us.

In all probability, if I asked you why you might be feeling depressed you might say...my boss is so demanding, or I hate my marriage, or my children are driving me crazy, or there's never enough money, or my best friend is dying of cancer, and so forth and so forth. The truth is that life is hard for most of us, but is has its marvelous side and comes with great rewards for those who persevere. Studies in stress tell us that if you're under too much of it, your serotonin levels can become depleted. Hence, you feel dismal and downcast. If you're struggling with feelings of sadness and hopelessness, you need to know about some simple measures you can take that have wonderful healing effects.

NOURISHING THE MIND

Besides keeping our bodies nutritionally sound and our environments conducive to good feelings, there are other activities we can incorporate into our lives that speed emotional healing and promote contentment. The whole concept behind naturopathy or natural medicine is to utilize a variety of natural healing techniques. Adding massage, breathing exercises, and meditation to herbal and nutritional medicine only enhances one's ability to get well. While these methods may be considered questionable by standard medical practitioners, they are far from new in their principles and applications. The link between the mind and wellness are drawn from the healing traditions of the India (Ayurvedic), China (Taoist), and Greece (Hippocratic).

Plautus once said that, "Only one man in ten knows himself." Consider some of the therapies listed as you read on. Experiment and try some of them on for size. Remember the admonition of Confucius: "The superior man will watch over himself when he is alone. He examines his heart, that there may be nothing wrong there, and that he may have no cause of dissatisfaction with himself"

BIOFEEDBACK

"The mind is restless, turbulent, obstinate and very strong. To subdue it is more difficult than controlling the wind, but it is possible by constant practice and attachment. He who strives by right means is assured of success."

Bhagavad Gita

Many experts in biofeedback firmly advocate its healing powers for depressive states of mind. Technically, biofeedback is based on the idea that if we can be taught to become aware of certain body functions, we can learn to control those functions. Biofeedback utilizes technical instruments which are used to monitor brain waves, blood pressure, skin temperature, heart rate, etc.

Through a feedback system, we can learn to actually control involuntary functions we normally have no idea how to affect. The ability to warm the hands, relieve muscle tension, lower blood pressure etc. are just a few techniques you can learn through biofeedback. Recent work with epileptics, who have been taught to ward of seizures through this type of self-awareness suggests that other neurological disorders may benefit from biofeedback. Some studies suggest that depressed people, like some epileptics, have a particular brain wave pattern.

The electrical activity of the brain can be classified into four types. Each correlates to a particular brain function and state of mental awareness.

ALPHA WAVES: Create a calming and clearing effect on the mind which is usually accompanied by a state of relaxation. Alpha waves can lead to more heightened levels of awareness.

BETA WAVES: Comprise the normal working rhythm of the brain. When beta waves become faster they reflect activity and stimuli. States of relaxation produce very little beta wave activity

THETA WAVES: Periods of meditation or creativity are usually characterized by theta waves.

DELTA WAVES: Delta waves are typical of sleep states but can be produced in some people when they are stimulated by a new idea or concept.

CAN DEPRESSION CREATE ITS OWN BRAIN WAVE?

Margaret Ayers, director of research at the Los Angeles-based Biofeedback and Advanced Therapy Institute found after five years of research, that primary depression without a manic component can manifest itself in a specific brain wave pattern. This pattern was characterized by slow waves and high voltage.

Ayers goal was to use biofeedback to change the biochemical profile of the brain, thereby affecting a psychological change. This particular approach is rather new in its concept. The notion of changing brain wave pattern to change emotional behavior has not been successfully done in the past. The concept, however, seems scientifically sound.

In 1975, it was discovered that brain waves recorded while epileptics slept revealed a distinct pattern of disorganized sleep and a tendency to motor twitching. By using biofeedback, seizures suffered by these epileptics were reduced. An unexpected result was that these individuals increased their ability to concentrate, had more energy, less aches and pains, and felt mentally reinvigorated.

In studying these findings, Ayers theorized that symptoms of depression could also be affected in the same way. She was able to fine tune the voltages of a biofeedback unit and enlisted the help of three depressed individuals to test her theories. What she discovered through their EEGs was that their waking brain wave patterns resembled those of the epileptics.

Using biofeedback techniques which train the patient to suppress unfavorable wave patterns, behavioral changes occurred. In other words, these depressed individuals succeeded in inhibiting the specific brain wave pattern that was associated with their depression. At the same time, they were able to produce another brain wave that suppressed feelings of depression.

All of these patients were examined by a clinical psychologist who was not told that they had undergone prior biofeedback treatment. The findings were all the same...the depression had been reversed. Like the epileptics, they also became more mentally alert, experienced a surge in energy and their mysterious aches and pains were greatly reduced or totally disappeared. As long as the brain wave pattern was changed, the beneficial results persisted.

WHAT ARE THE MECHANICS OF BIOFEEDBACK?

How does biofeedback for depression work? Surface electrodes are placed on the scalp on a one inch strip which runs from ear to ear. These electrodes are hooked to a Neuroanalyzer unit, which is connected to a polygraph, which records filtered brain wave patterns on paper.

In biofeedback, the patient experiences an EEG feedback. In other words, positive rewards for achieving certain brain wave patterns are given in the form of an orange light, a certain digital number, or a beeping tone. These rewards serve as positive reinforcements for the elimination of negative frequency bands. A red light indicates that the desired brain wave alteration is not occurring. The treatment gets progressively harder in order to more fully train an individual in achieving control over his or her physiology.

Ayers believes that when the brain becomes depressed it gets in a rut, meaning that it doesn't know how to correct itself. Based on this theory, she believes biofeedback can be tremendously beneficial in guiding the brain back to a normal state. The brain, in its attempt to achieve a homeostasis or normal biochemical balance is capable of producing high frequency brain waves which suppress slow wave activity. Her findings show that biofeedback teaches the brain to accomplish this in such a way that both brain wave patterns eventually disappear.

The normal period of time required for biofeedback therapy for depression is between two and three months. Typically a biofeedback training program consists of ten hour long, weekly sessions. The research findings we have just talked about imply that biofeedback may provide a noninvasive treatment for depression, designed to implement a learned brain wave pattern. It may offer a viable, long-term alternative for people who suffer from depression.

The possible benefits of biofeedback for depression should be investigated. Like so many other treatments discussed in this book, the ability to heal oneself may exist in unexpected therapies and activities. Biofeedback has been successfully used for treating migraine headaches, hypertension, Raynaud's disease and stress related disorders. In addition, using learned techniques such as warming your hands can help to relieve arthritis, angina, irritable bowel syndrome, diabetes, menopausal symptoms and impotence.

ADDED BENEFITS OF BIOFEEDBACK
FOR DEPRESSED INDIVIDUALS

Elmer E. Green Ph.D who founded the Biofeedback and Psychophysiology Center of the Menninger Foundation believes that any chronic condition that has a psychosomatic link can be treated with biofeedback. One of the most promising aspects of biofeedback for depressed people is that the realization that one can control what are considered involuntary processes of the body. This creates a feeling of empowerment. This notion of self-mastery is crucial for anyone who is depressed, because depression snatches away control. Biofeedback enables people to treat themselves in a way no one ever thought possible.

Many insurance companies now cover biofeedback and many hospitals have practitioners trained in the technique. This fact alone has elevated the status of biofeedback within conventional medicine. If you tell your doctor you're interested in exploring biofeedback, you might even get a positive response. People who respond best to biofeedback are those who have a strong ability to visualize and are tenacious.

MEDITATION

"There is one art of which man should master, the art of reflection."

Samuel Coleridge

Like so many ancient healing practices, meditation has often been overlooked as a marvelous healing tool. Being able to meditate teaches us how to access deeper states of consciousness. Meditation can effectively block out the negative thought patterns which threaten to destroy us during a bout with depression. Meditation helps us connect with our unconscious minds. In so doing, feelings of spiritual awareness and tranquility can be produced.

When you meditate, marked changes in your physiology occur, as well as a clarification of thought processes. Dr. Benson in his book *The Relaxation Response* demonstrates that meditation can normalize blood pressure, lower pulse rate, decrease the levels of stress hormones in the blood and produce changes in brain-wave patterns.

HOW TO MEDITATE

There are several methods of meditation, all designed to achieve the same end. You can focus on a symbolic sound or mantra, a single image or mandala, such as a flame, or even become acutely aware of the rhythmic patterns of your own breathing. Any of these methods produce a deep, calm, restful trance-like state which frees them mind from anxiety and confusion.

Concerning meditation, Bernie Seigel, M.D. in his book *Love, Medicine and Miracles* says, "I know of no other single activity that by itself can produce such a great improvement in the quality of life." Isn't it a shame that something as beneficial as meditation is not routinely taught in our society. Again, ancient civilizations were more knowledgeable about the value of so many natural healing therapies that have managed to elude our highly educated modern culture.

It's been exciting to see, however, a new awareness of the healing powers of meditation and visualization on disease. Meditation does indeed alter brain function, endocrine function and the immune system, three areas which are intimately linked with depressive illness. If you're down, you think a certain way. In other words you get into the habit of continually bombarding your mind with pessimistic ideas like...I'll never get well, I hate people, life is a cosmic joke, there's no future for me, or I don't belong here. When you feel down, you have a tendency to complain and become overly critical of everything and everyone.

SCIENTIFIC ASPECTS OF MEDITATION

Scientific research has proven that thoughts and feelings affect neurotransmitter production. Habitually engaging in negative, anxious or hostile thoughts can alter the chemical makeup of the brain resulting in behavioral changes. A steady diet of undesirable images or thoughts determines how we feel and what choices we make. It is for this very reason that the impact of violence and sex in movies and television on America's youth is of such concern. Our minds are impressionable and vulnerable to manipulation.

Learning how to effectively meditate will not be easy. Western culture doesn't teach us how to engage in these types of activities. In other words, we'll have to fight our overwhelming resistance to clearing our consciousness. Buddhists refer to the untrained mind as a "drunken monkey stung by a bee." This sounds like a pretty accurate description of my own state of mind.

Because true meditation is difficult to cultivate, make sure you use it only as a supplement to nutritional and exercise changes. There are instructional books available on meditation. Most of them suggest sitting down, with your back straight either on the floor or on a chair. Your aim will be to direct all your attention to a particular object such as a flickering flame. Your mind will inevitably wander from your chosen object and so you will re-direct your attention back. You will have to do this over and over again until you master the ability to prohibit distractive thoughts from entering your consciousness.

Learning how to meditate takes a lot of discipline and may prove too challenging for someone who is struggling with extreme mental fatigue. The concept behind meditation is unquestionably sound and certainly holds promise as a therapy for depression. Remember, that so often we look outside of ourselves for the answers or the solutions to personal dilemmas. Learning to meditate can sharpen and empower the strengths we all have that come from within, rather than without. Regarding the dreariness and desolation of depression, Camus put it best: "In the midst of winter, I finally learned that there was in me an invincible summer."

BREATHING

"Everything intercepts us from ourselves."
Ralph Waldo Emerson

Breathing exercises can be surprisingly effective at dispelling mental fatigue, relaxing the nervous system and creating a sense of tranquility. Everyday, at the same time, or when you feel particularly unable to cope, concentrate on your breathing. Put everything else out of your mind and become acutely conscious of each and every breath you take.

Several yoga books contain good breathing exercises, however any good system works on the same principles. Most involve positioning the tongue against the back of the teeth throughout the exercise. You begin by first exhaling completely through the mouth. Making a hissing sound can help to expedite a thorough expulsion of air in a slow and controlled manner. Next, you begin to inhale through your nose with your mouth closed while you are counting to five in your head. Now, hold your breath for approximately 6 to 7 seconds. Begin to exhale slowly through your mouth, making the same hissing sound and count to 7 in your mind. At this point, take another breath and repeat the same sequence of events. You can do this three to four times.

Controlled breathing exercises such as this one have a wonderful tranquilizing effect and should be done on a daily basis, or as many times as your feel you need them. Some experts not only recommend using breathing techniques such as this one to dissipate stress or anxiety, but for insomnia as well. Feeling relaxed and tranquil are the results of learning how to use breathing to your advantage. When you're depressed, you know how difficult it can be to do something as simple as relax.

There are several other ways to facilitate a relaxed state. Yoga, as mentioned earlier offers an excellent program of body exercises designed to promote relaxation. If you want to try yoga, you'll have more success if you sign up for a class and do it under the supervision of a professional instructor.

Manipulating your breathing can exert a strong influence on the mind, the body and you moods. In many respects, breathing exercises are nothing more than another form of meditation. Something as simple as the conscious regulation of breath can initiate a number of desirable effects. It's easy enough to do and incorporate into your life. I have personally found that it is an invaluable way to dispel the kind of mounting stress we often encounter in the work place or in dealing with family stressors.

Controlled breathing acts like a natural tranquilizer. Whenever you feel like tension is mounting, kick into action. Just the fact that a shift in your consciousness occurs during this type of exercise can enable you to disconnect from negative thought patterns and achieve relaxation. Keep in mind that it is normal to feel a little lightheaded when you first start.

MASSAGE THERAPY

The human body should be considered as several interconnected systems that make up a whole. When you see the human body in this way, the potential healing effects of therapies designed to work one part of the body to affect another become understandable. Manipulating or rubbing the deep tissues of our musculature can stimulate us both physically and mentally. Applying touch or pressure to certain muscle groups through massage therapy can help to restore function and surprisingly, actually improve mental outlook.

There are several schools of massage from the Chinese and Japanese to the Swedish. American Indians also used massage to achieve relaxation through what was more vigorously brushing the body rather than actually rubbing it.

When it comes to depression the value of massage therapy is contained in the idea that when nerves are stimulated through muscle groups, feelings of well being and exhilaration can be facilitated. Being touched is a basic human need and some experts believe that when you're depressed, that need is intensified.

Massage therapy executed with essential oils is superbly relaxing. Ask around and make an appointment with a skilled and reputable therapist. The money involved for massage therapy is well worth the rewards and is really quite inexpensive considering what we willingly spend on manicures, perms, golf etc. This type of massage takes advantage of not only muscle manipulation but aromatherapy as well.

Feeling anxious, restless, irritable, sleepless or sad can all be reflected in your posture and the state of your muscles. Tense individuals who suffer from chronic stiff necks know all about this phenomenon. We unconsciously manifest our emotional states in our musculature, much more so than most of us can imagine.

Massage therapy with essential oils affords its recipient the opportunity to relax these muscles and to clear the mind while doing so. The penetrability and aroma of essential oils enhances the benefits of massage. Continual rubbing and kneading of not only the neck, shoulders and back, but of the forehead, face, chin, top of the hands, chest, and feet stimulates nerve endings and boosts peripheral circulation. Scalp massages are especially good for both physical and mental fatigue and can help to restore feelings of energy and elevate moods.

TYPES OF MASSAGE

Taoist masters used a massage system called chi lei jong which concentrates on massaging the abdomen. It is particularly good for redirecting blood flow and stimulating the lymphatic system. It can be self-administered and should be looked into.

Swedish massage, which usually comprises several basic strokes applied to soft body tissues can tranquilize the nervous system. This vigorous form of massage stimulates circulation and can relieve tension. It is also used to help individuals cope with various emotional problems. Apparently, the very act of massage can help bring emotions to the surface.

Granted, the effects of any massage or aromatherapy are only temporary. Done on a regular basis, however, their cumulative benefits should not be minimized. If you can't afford regular massages, invest in a good, electrical massage unit. New models include shiatsu massage units which apply deep rhythmic massage. I use one of these units myself and if you're alone a lot, it can be a real blessing. When I get overly tense or just need to unwind and clear my mind, I use the machine for ten minutes. The effects are quite refreshing. My attitude invariably improves after a treatment.

PROGRESSIVE RELAXATION

This particular technique produces a feeling of relaxation and is especially good for treating insomnia and anxiety. The exercises are easy and are based on a simple procedure of alternating between a state of tension and relaxation in the muscles. Initially, you contract a muscle as hard as you can for a period of two seconds, after which you totally relax that muscle. You repeat this exercise for another muscle and then another, until your entire body falls into a state of sublime relaxation.

Lie on your back and take two deep, controlled breaths before you start. Starting with the muscles of the face and neck and then progressing to the upper arms, chest and back is the usual sequence. The process is repeated for the abdomen, buttocks, thighs, calves and feet. You may want to start by clenching your teeth and squeezing your eyes and work down to making tight fists, and pulling your stomach muscles in toward your spinal column. Make sure that you go completely limp after each contraction.

If you need to, repeat the whole process again and then lie perfectly still with your eyes closed. Listen to the natural rhythm of your breathing and concentrate on remaining free from tension of any kind. Some experts recommend taping sequential step by step instructions for this exercise on a cassette and playing it right after you get into bed. This particular method can be used at work or during the day if you feel yourself tensing up. Progressive relaxation can be done in any position.

You can train yourself to become very adept at progressive relaxation. The idea behind this technique is that by contrasting the differences between tension and relaxation, the latter is intensified. In time, you'll have the order in which you tense and relax muscle groups down, and the exercise will become automatic. The following muscle groups are recommended:

Forehead: wrinkle your forehead and relax

Mouth: open your mouth as wide as it goes and then bit down and clench your jaw (not too tightly or you could damage your jaw joint), then relax.

Shoulders: lift your shoulders to your ears, hold them there, then relax.

Chest: inhale and fill your lungs completely, hold for 3 seconds then slowly exhale and relax.

Arms: clench your fists and contract your arm muscles hard, then relax.

Stomach: bulge your stomach out as far as it can go then pull in it as hard as you can then relax.

Back: arch your spine as high as you can get it of the floor, hold it then relax.

Hips and upper legs: Rock your knees and exert pressure on your heels, digging them into the floor then relax.

Lower legs and feet: Lightly curl your toes while you extend your legs out, lift them off the floor, keeping them stiff, then relax.

Progressive relaxation is a marvelous way to unwind and combat the kind of stress and anxiety that would hurt our ability to feel tranquil or to sleep well. Remember to concentrate solely on what's happening with each muscle group and don't let your mind wander. Part of the reason that so many of us can't relax or get to sleep is that we let our attention slip into dismal thought patterns that directly impact a number of biological systems with negative input.

MUSIC THERAPY

"Music is the art of the prophets, the only art that can calm the agitations of the soul."

Martin Luther

What we hear can profoundly affect the state of our nervous system. Ask anyone who lives with a teenager about the influence of loud, hard rock music on most adults and they'll passionately tell you; it can make them feel like they're losing their minds.

Music directly or indirectly impacts the subconscious mind. It can create feelings of tension and irritability, or of peace and serenity. Drum rhythms and ritual sound repetitions prompt sensations of ecstacy, mysticism, sexual excitement and hypnotic states.

Noises that commonly fill our environment can subconsciously determine our state of mind. Although most of us are unaware of background noises, they can subtly color the way we see things and how we feel. I have found that sometimes my subconscious perception of TV dialogue playing in another room can make me feel jumpy and progressively tense if I am reading or working at the computer.

If you suffer from depression it is important to choose specific kinds of sound for your environment. The choice is individual, however, certain effects seem universally beneficial. Slow moving classical music, soft jazz, certain nature sounds like rain falling or the sound of a water fall usually calm and pacify. On the other hand, strong, rhythmic drumbeats, high pitched noises and loud fast moving music can grate on our nerves and create emotional disturbance.

MUSIC AND PHYSIOLOGY

In hospitals, relaxing music has been shown to actually decrease blood pressure in coronary patients. The most effective type of music seems to have a tempo of around 70 to 80 beats per minute which is almost the same as the average pulse rate.

In depressive illness, music therapy serves to break down the walls that can make you feel isolated from the rest of the world. It can, in some cases, enable a depressed individual to feel more talkative or even outgoing. Music has been used more extensively over the last few years to not only stimulate the nervous system of depressed people, but to draw autistics and schizophrenics out of their private worlds.

Just because a selection of music seems calm and mellow doesn't mean its desirable for melancholia. Some kinds of music are intrinsically sad and full of pathos and should be avoided. The soundtrack to Schindler's list is full of profound sorrow and should be avoided if you're fighting depression. Baroque instrumental music has been used in Europe for its ability to create a sensation of calm well being. Some studies have shown that when you listen to this type of music, your heartbeat will eventually synchronize itself with the musical beat and relaxation will occur.

Other kinds of desirable music and sounds include gentle ballads, classical guitar, spiritual compositions, waves pounding, bird songs and night crickets.

SLEEP

*"We are such stuff as dreams are made on, and our little
life is rounded with sleep."*

William Shakespeare

Despite the fact that we sleep for almost half of our lives, sleep and
its relationship to health has been surprisingly neglected by physicians
and scientists. It's been only within the last two decades that the effects
of sleep disorders have been addressed. Evidence supports the fact that
anyone of these sleep disorders can exert a profound, detrimental effect
upon both our physical and mental states.

Unquestionably, an innate relationship exists between depression
and sleep. Four out of five people who become depressed view bedtime
with dread. What should be a time to peacefully rest and rejuvenate
becomes a period of tossing and turning, characterized by obsessive,
negative thoughts. The simple ability to relax and fall asleep peacefully
becomes almost impossible for many depressed individuals. Moreover,
even if they get to sleep, they frequently awake and fill that wakefulness
with distressing and troubling thoughts.

What do depressed people think about. Anything and everything
that is gloomy, scary or self-defeating. I have had some experience with
troubled sleep. I wake up at 3:30 AM and I worry about money,
earthquakes, getting fat, being alone, comets hitting the earth, my
children's health, and the seeming finality of death, just to name a few
choice subjects. When this happens, sleep vanishes and the anxiety I
experience will usually escalate until the early morning hours. If I do
get some pre-dawn rest, it's minimal and I wake up feeling exhausted
and grumpy.

You'll probably agree that these kinds of thought patterns can
become exacerbated during periods of sleeplessness and usually aren't
based on reality. As most of you know, lying in the dark can intensify
fearful and apprehensive feelings and make everything seem a hundred
times worse than it really is. Thankfully, the arrival of day frequently
helps to dispel many of our night terrors. On the other hand, in cases of
severe depression, the torture can continue.

ALL SLEEP ISN'T NECESSARILY GOOD SLEEP

Undoubtedly, sleep disturbances can both cause depressive illness, or result from its presence. Some scientists believe that the wrong kind of sleep initiates depression, a condition which results from an imbalance of brain chemistry. They suggest that the chemical changes which occur in the brain during sleep may have a direct bearing on the nerves and neurotransmitters that produce depression.

Perhaps this finally explains the existence of "morning people." Surely there must be a biological reason why some of us wake up grumpy, moody and irritable while others are prone to singing and whistling. The notion that sleeping in and of itself may not be enough to promote good mood is worth investigating. Perhaps, the kind of sleep we get is just as important as how long we sleep. Most people who feel depressed not only experience shortened intervals of sleep, any sleep they do get is poor.

It's common knowledge that unsatisfactory sleep can cause impaired alertness which frequently results in accidents of all kinds. Some experts believe that American operates on a sleep deficit which goes unrecognized as a major causal factor in many types of erratic behavior. Most of us go to bed too late, sleep faultily or take hypnotic drugs which make us feel unrested and mentally fogged. In a study on sleep deprivation, forty percent of the subjects tested were found to be "pathologically sleepy."

Clearly, much of the evidence in this book supports that fact that disturbed brain biochemistry can be responsible for nighttime as well as daytime mind sets. If you consistently wake up early and fall into anxious thought patterns, you won't be able to sleep well. Consequently, you may feel like you haven't slept at all. Sleeping poorly should not be considered a normal condition and almost always signals the presence of another disorder. This is especially true for depression.

REM SLEEP AND DEPRESSIVE ILLNESS

Research has found that most depressed individuals enter REM sleep more rapidly than normal. This particular phenomenon is also typical of people suffering from schizophrenia, anorexia, mania, obsessive-compulsive disorder and some personality disorders. Interestingly, a whole host of psychiatric diseases manifest disturbed sleep patterns. Anxiety and dementia result in decreased delta waves during sleep, and panic disorders produce continually interrupted and decreased sleep. What research findings suggest is that if you're suffering from depression, even when you do sleep, you may not be experiencing true rest. Disruptions in REM sleep are clearly a marker of behavioral disorders, and attest to the complex interrelationship of all body systems.

Some studies have shown that by depriving a person from achieving REM sleep for an extended period of time, various psychotic conditions result, including severe depressive illness. The fact that a continual lack of quality sleep can actually accumulate over time is a concept most of us are unaware of. In time, this sleep debt can gradually result in subtle, unexplained symptoms. Interrupting the way the brain normally falls asleep, stays asleep, and wakes up can create a sleep deficit.

If you take any kind of drug, you may be significantly compromising the quality of your sleep. Sedatives, stimulants like caffeine, anticonvulsants and antihistamines are just a few of the many chemical agents that interfere with normal sleep patterns causing daytime fatigue. It's also important to know that if you are withdrawing from any of these drugs, your sleep may be altered for several weeks as your body adjusts to the withdrawal of these chemical agents from the bloodstream.

Sleep disruption is like depression is that it can be initiated by so many hidden factors. Smoking and obesity can affect respiration, which can result in sleep apnea. Sleep apnea refers to a condition of abnormal breathing or snoring which can actually deprive brain cells from adequate oxygen. A repeated lack of oxygen to brain tissue can result in mental fogginess, forgetfulness or emotional stupor. Exposure to polluted air, water, certain organic compounds, and heavy metals can also intrude on and alter normal sleep. In addition, food allergies are notorious for causing insomnia or restless sleep, especially in children.

SEROTONIN, SLEEP AND DEPRESSION

It almost seems redundant at this point in our discussion to bring up the "S" word again. Serotonin not only assists in initiating REM sleep but has to be present in certain levels to adequately maintain REM sleep. Scientists have recently concluded that serotonin levels are crucial determinants in both the sleeping and waking cycles. Clinical depression can be seen in most cases, as a lack of adequate serotonin levels in brain tissue.

The amino acid, tryptophan was commonly used as a natural treatment for insomnia. Before it was taken off the market, tryptophan was successfully used to induce normal sleep. The fact that tryptophan is a precursor to serotonin which also helps to define our moods and attitudes must be considered here. The serotonin component of both sleep and depression reiterates how intimately linked the two states are. Artificial manipulation of serotonin through chemical agents can actually interfere with sleep. It's fascinating to learn that antidepressant drugs of the SSRIs variety like Prozac actually inhibit REM sleep due to their unnatural action on serotonin levels. A common side-effect of Prozac is the inability to sleep well.

Serotonin is also a crucial neurotransmitter in the raphe system of the brain, which is intimately linked to the sleeping state. If serotonin levels are abnormally low, sleeping intervals decrease. In other words, you wake up before you're supposed to.

Another reason why you feel so lousy mentally when you don't sleep well is that the cells of the nervous system are regenerated and rebuilt structurally during REM sleep. If you don't get enough REM sleep, protein production in the CNS is inhibited, thereby preventing the normal restoration of cells required to keep us mentally healthy.

The message here is apparent. We need a certain amount of REM sleep to feel happy and healthy. Ironically, many drugs, some of which are used to help induce sleep or counteract depression can actually interfere with or diminish REM sleep. To make matters even more confusing, disrupted sleep can cause depression and depression can cause disrupted sleep. Finding out which came first could prove difficult. In any event, just knowing that serotonin levels are so crucial to proper REM sleep, sheds new insight into sleep and its intrinsic relationship with depression.

Examining brain wave patterns of depressed individuals who are sleeping may also be valuable in assessing the potential of therapies like biofeedback for insomnia and depression. If brain wave patterns in depressed people can be identified, then learning to control these patterns may be possible.

SEDATIVE DRUGS, ARTIFICIALLY INDUCED
SLEEP AND DEPRESSION

If you have trouble sleeping, really make an effort to forgo the drug route and concentrate on relaxation techniques and natural therapies. If possible, avoid the temptation to use sedatives or other sleep promoting drugs. They are highly addictive and only serve to make you feel even more tired and depressed. This type of artificial sleep is not true, restful sleep. On the contrary, sedative medications can make you feel hungover and can aggravate depressive illness.

Every year, up to ten million people in the United States use prescription drugs to get to sleep. Benzodiazepines can produce a variety of undesirable side-effects including lethargy, amnesia, memory impairment, nervousness and aggressiveness. These drugs act on brain chemistry, therefore affecting behavior as well.

I would think it safe to assume, that even if you're depressed and suffering from insomnia, o 98.f the worst things you could do to yourself is to add benzodiazepines to your system. This family of hypnotic drugs which include Halcion, Valium, Librium Ativan, Dalmane, and Clonopin to mention only a few, have been shown to increase feelings of depression and even prompt suicidal thinking.

The typical scenario goes something like this: You can't sleep, so you take a sleeping pill, which disrupts normal sleep patterns by suppressing REM sleep. REM sleep is the best kind. During REM sleep your body repairs itself and dreams are generated. Because you will be deprived of REM sleep by your sleeping pill, you'll wake up more tired than you were before you went to sleep. To make matters worse, if you try to stop taking these pills after long term use, you can experience severe withdrawal symptoms which include anxiety, seizures, hallucinations, panic, insomnia, memory loss and depression. So, you go back on them.

Before you initiate the vicious cycle of artificial sedation, try relaxation techniques, dietary changes, amino acids and herbs. Getting a good night's sleep is wonderful medicine and obviously helps us feel refreshed.

While it is typical for depressed people to sleep poorly, for some people with melancholia, oversleeping is the rule. Hypersomnia refers to the need for more than a normal amount of sleep, and can also occur when you feel depressed, especially in seasonal mood disorders. For more information regarding hypersomnia, see the section of Seasonal Affective Disorder. Keep in mind that getting too much sleep can make you feel as unrested as getting too little. Our biological clocks usually determine the optimal amount of sleep we need to feel good. When we sleep too little or too much, that clock is off, and nine times out of ten, it's due to a neurochemical disruption.

Regardless of whether you're undersleeping or oversleeping, if your depression continues to worsen, your sleep disorders will intensify. Again, as in the case of mood, the connection between brain amines like tryptophan and sleeping are complex. One thing is certain, when brain biochemistry is off, sleep is bound to be affected in some way. Remember also that just getting to sleep and staying asleep doesn't always provide the body with the ideal time to regenerate itself. Using prescription hypnotic drugs attests to this fact.

WAKE UP SLOWLY

How we wake up from sleep is also crucial in determining our mental attitude. If we consistently experience interrupted sleep, we may be perpetrating and encouraging more depression. This type of sleep pattern, if continued indefinitely can greatly precipitate melancholia and promote restlessness. Dr. Deepak Chopra M.D. in his book *Quantum Healing* points out that humans need to wake up from sleep through a series of timed signals that progress from mild to strong. He stresses that ideally, to go from the biochemistry of sleep to the biochemistry of wakefulness, the transition should be gradual.

To the contrary, most of us are abruptly woken out of a dead sleep by a blaring alarm which jars our brains out of its state of rest. Likewise, if you wake up in the middle of your sleep cycle and disrupt the normal pattern of sleep, you feel groggy, moody and irritable during the day.

Sleep improvement is often the first sign that depression is lifting. As you get well, you will fall asleep faster and begin to sleep through the night. In conjunction with better sleep, your appetite will improve, and your spirits will rise. The domino effect here is a desirable one, with each positive biochemical change initiating another.

SLEEP DEPRIVATION

One, somewhat controversial natural method for controlling some depression is found in sleep deprivation. This prohibition of sleep does not refer to the random kind which continually inhibits REM sleep, but is controlled and individually programed. This particular treatment assumes that depression has a tendency to put the brain to sleep in an unnatural way. By programming periods of wakefulness, the brain, in some instances become stimulated. As a result, mood and behavior improve.

Some new studies at the National Institute of Mental Health in Bethesda, Maryland have shown that sleep deprivation may actually help some people who are depressed feel better. This technique is based on the fact that in some cases, the controlled absence of sleep may serve to snap some people out of a depressive state.

Surprisingly, these studies have found that staying up all night for these individuals promotes cheerfulness, conversation and light-hearted feelings in even seriously depressed people. Because the depressive illness returns when these individuals resume their normal sleeping patterns, a system of partial sleep in which patients intersperse nights where they sleep for only five hours with normal sleeping hours have been recommended.

Interestingly, one theory as to why this works with certain people is that sleep deprivation can stimulate TSH from a sluggish thyroid gland. The connection between inadequate amounts of thyroid hormone and depression are addressed in an earlier chapter. A controlled lack of sleep can actually help to restore cortisol and TSH to normal levels, thus improving mood. It would seem plausible that anyone responding to this type of therapy, should have their thyroid checked.

Partial-sleep deprivation therapy has worked for 60 percent of patients suffering from major depression. It must be stressed here that this type of treatment is not for everyone suffering from depression and should only be done under the supervision of an expert. Sleep deprivation can be dangerous and can precipitate erratic behavior.

Some doctors have also used sleep deprivation as a preventive measure for people who have a history of periodic bouts with depression. This treatment involved staying up for 36 hours once a week and should be done only under the care of a doctor or health practitioner.

Another interesting aspect of sleep deprivation is that sometimes it works when antidepressant drugs fail. Like other natural therapies, no significant side-effects have been observed, nevertheless, you need to find out if you're a candidate for this radical form of treatment. For many people, the therapy has proven effective.

The sleep connection to depression is another piece of evidence that brain biochemistry is intrinsically linked to how we eat and how we sleep. If you want more information on the partial-sleep program contact Dr. Thomas Wehr and Dr. David A. Sack at the National Institute of Mental Health, in Bethesda, Maryland.

SPIRITUAL HEALING

"For he will command His angels concerning you to guard you in all your ways; they will lift you up in their hands, so that you will not strike your foot against a stone."

Psalms 91:11,12

Thank goodness that drawing on the powers of heaven is not the taboo subject it used to be. As we approach a new millennia, great segments of our population are openly admitting their innate need for spiritual nourishment. The soul has been badly neglected and even abused by our societal focus on money, power and gain. Within academic and intellectual circles, the worth and value of religion or spiritual acknowledgement are usually scoffed at and cast aside. In our efforts to employ the scientific method to validate anything and everything, we have forgotten the ultimate healing power of spiritual medicine.

Our hesitance to include the viability of supernatural help in enhancing the healing of disease into scholastic discussions has often resulted in the complete disregard of its potential. Why are we afraid to encourage the incorporation of spiritual helps as a way to get well? Perhaps, people will think we're a bit eccentric, or maybe even a little strange. Lily Tomlin has jokingly said, "Why is it when we talk to God we are said to be praying, and when God talks to us we're said to be schizophrenic?

If we are battling with depression, a pernicious enemy from within, we need to trust more in powers unseen to fortify ourselves. In so doing, we can truly discover who we really are and our immeasurable worth as living souls. Goethe said, "As soon as you trust yourself you will know how to live." Trust your ability to get in tune with your spiritual self. Trust that there is a loving God who is aware of your struggles. Ask for help and expect to receive it. Man was created that he might have joy, not despair.

If you decide to try natural therapies to help you get well, remember that unlike the scientific community, you can expect miracles. C.S.

Lewis expresses it beautifully, "By miracles, we don't mean contradictions to nature. We mean that left to her own resources, she could never produce them." Employ the power of prayer to facilitate the miracle of wellness for yourself.

When you rise in the morning, pray. Express gratitude for life and thanks for the opportunity to be alive then let our Creator know what your specific needs are. Ask in faith, believing that you are loved and that your life is precious. One study called "The Efficacy of Prayer" by Plant J. Collipp M.D. suggested that prayer does indeed have value in the treatment of disease. Dr. Collipp states, "Among the plethora of modern drugs, and the increasing ingenuity of our surgeons, it seems inappropriate that our medical literature contains so few studies on our oldest and, who knows, perhaps most successful form of therapy [i.e., prayer]."

Even Carl Jung, in his treatise *Modern Man in Search of a Soul* remained profoundly dissatisfied with conventional therapies for the mentally ill. His interest in the metaphysical or the supernatural grew from his observation that Freud's methods of treating people with psychological disorders did not seem to work if they were over the age of 35. He confides, "It is safe to say that every one of them fell ill because he had lost that which the living religions of every age have given to their followers, and none of them has been really healed who did not regain his religious outlook."

If you don't have any spiritual roots, cultivate some. Seek out God and learn to have faith. Never underestimate the power of love which helps us to break out of our sometimes obsessive preoccupation with ourselves. Eric Fromm has said, "In addition to faith, we must possess courage, the willingness to take a risk, even to experience pain and disappointment..."

Know that your life has meaning. Believing that we're here strictly as the result of a cosmic accident is the most depressing thing I've ever heard. Lewis Thomas tells us that statistically, the probability of any one of us being here is so small that you'd think the mere fact of existing would keep us all in contented dazzlement of surprise. Sadly, as humans, we don't react that way. We routinely become accustomed to miraculous events. Worse yet, most of us don't view our own existence as the ultimate miracle, worthy of wild celebration.

Certainly many of us have been gravely disappointed in our lives. Unquestionably, many of us are confused...troubled by issues of sexuality, intimacy, moral values, marital discord and the search for meaning. Our society as a whole has lost its spiritual faith and replaced it with cynicism instead. The results have been catastrophic. The disintegration of all kinds of love, familial, marital etc., has resulted in the deterioration of our love for God.

So many of us feel as though we've become estranged from our God, especially if we feel depressed. When we let that happen, we become unfamiliar with the language of the spirit. By so doing, we deprive ourselves of a marvelous healing dimension. We've talked about getting in touch with our inner selves through meditation, relaxation etc. Prayer is very rarely suggested in most self-help literature, an error which constitutes nothing less than a gross oversight. How many of us can say that we have tried to cultivate a personal rapport with our Creator? Even the current religious resurgence many of us see all around us can never take the place of the private cultivation of a deep, intimate relationship with God. All the psychoanalysis and all the antidepressants in the world can never heal us so completely.

THE VERDICT'S IN:
The Serotonin Did It.

If there exists in medical annals a disease which proves the delicate interconnecting relationships between the mind and the body, it's depression. The most stunning discovery of the research complied for this book is the fact that even the most minor disruption of brain chemistry can result in a "blue" feeling. Moreover, what causes these disruptions can be something as overtly insignificant as a lack of sunlight or a subtle enzyme disfunction in the brain.

The findings of each and every section of this book have pointed to the same message over and over. Serotonin levels in the brain, which are extremely important in the determination of mood, can be decreased by a number of seemingly unrelated factors. Amazingly, these factors can bounce off of each other making the question of what causes what first very difficult to assess. There can be no question, however, that everything we do, eat, and expose ourselves to can affect brain biochemistry and alter mood.

Let's tell a perfectly terrible story that to our dismay, sounds vaguely familiar. We'll call it:

THE SEROTONIN CAPER

Your life is stressful so you eat snack food on the run...which makes you become deficient in B-vitamins...which lowers serotonin levels in your brain...which makes you feel tired...which makes you reach for caffeine...which can interfere with normal brain chemistry...which makes you feel depressed...which makes you lack energy...which makes you reach for sugar which can make your glucose levels unstable...which can adversely affect serotonin levels and deplete B-vitamins...which makes you feel depressed...which makes you hibernate...which makes you sunshine deprived...which makes your serotonin go down...which makes you feel depressed...which makes you inactive...which makes you gain weight, which makes you take diet pills...which promotes low serotonin levels...which makes you lack energy...which makes you more sedentary...which makes you constipated...which makes you feel depressed...which aggravates PMS symptoms...which causes an estrogen imbalance...which lowers serotonin levels...which makes you get less REM sleep...which makes you take a sleeping pill...which makes you feel depressed...which makes you reach for a drink...which depletes B-vitamins...which lowers serotonin...which makes you feel depressed...and so on and so on and so on...

If we've learned anything about serotonin, it's that we must become acutely aware of how our lifestyle choices affect our biochemistry. If we want to be happy, we have to be smart about our choices. Most importantly, if we've gotten ourselves into a vicious feedback loop such as the one described above, we have to break the very cycle we often promote through our own bad habits.

GAME PLAN:
Overall Strategy for treating and preventing depression

"Chance never helps those who do not help themselves"

Sophocles

Okay, are you ready to commit to making the inside you and your outside world as antidepressant as possible? There is so much that all of us can do to scare the goblins of depression away and get on with the business of living. Hellen Keller put it beautifully when she said, "the world is very full of suffering, it is also full of the overcoming of it." Even in the midst of your darkest winter, you can find your invincible summer.

Let's be frank, it's going to be difficult. Life has a way of being very unaccommodating and when you're depressed, it seems to have a personal vendetta against you and only you. Typically, manuals on depression advocate a number of positive thinking exercises to improve your mental attitude and your perception of reality. Learning how to release anger, or to confront problems is good, however, in most cases, in and of itself won't cure you of a good ol fashioned chemically induced depression.

When all is said and done, you need to incorporate tangible and practical suggestions for relieving and preventing depression in combination with spiritual exercises such as mediation and prayer. The following guide has been derived from information discussed in this book. Look it over and then incorporate its suggestions into the fabric of your very lives.

The tools are at your disposal. You can and will feel happy again, contented, fulfilled. It's not something that you have to feverishly pursue. It will just happen. Edith Wharton once said facetiously, " If only we'd stop trying to be happy, we could have a pretty good time." In times of depression, however, we have to sometimes work at becoming happy again. All of us need to have a reason to get up in the morning. To find that reason, we must live by a set of guiding principles. If you've lost your map, get another one and always remember that the human body, when it is nourished and cared for has an absolutely miraculous ability to heal itself. Keep the words of Jean Bodin first and foremost on your mind as you plan your strategy, "The good life is the healthful life, the merry life. Life is health, joy, laughter."

HOW TO CREATE AN ANTIDEPRESSIVE EXTERNAL ENVIRONMENT

- Fill your environment with wonderful aromas by using light bulb rings and essential fragrant oils. Coming home to a house filled with the smell of cinnamon can go a long way to promote a sense of tranquility and well being
- If the news depresses you, cancel your newspaper and watch a video instead of the ten o'clock news broadcast.
- Get plenty of sunlight. If sunlight is not available, obtain adequate sources of strong artificial light. Install a skylight or invest in a light box.
- Surround yourself with plenty of green plants, flowers and other growing things. Cultivate a garden.
- Play uplifting music that perks up the spirit and makes you feel optimistic.
- Get a pet.

GOOD HABITS TO GET INTO

- Get outside and exercise on a regular basis. If the weather is disagreeable, make sure you exercise indoors. Invest in a piece of equipment you are most likely to use. Treadmills are usually very good and are utilized more that fancy contraptions that cost a fortune.
- When you get home, pop in a soothing and mood elevating CD (Baroque strings, Mozart, Kenny G etc.).
- Practice controlled breathing exercises at least once a day.
- Get a weekly massage using essential oils or use a home unit.
- Use daily meditation or breathing exercises to center your life and prevent mood swings.
- Use progressive relaxation techniques to unwind.
- Take a hot bath with aromatic oils every night 30 minutes before retiring.
- Consistently cultivate a spiritual philosophy centered around a

loving God.
* Pray always.

NUTRITIONAL GUIDELINES

* Eliminate all forms of caffeine, alcohol, nicotine and any other unnecessary prescription or over-the-counter drugs
* Cut down or eliminate sugar all together from your diet. Eat a diet high in raw fruits, vegetable, whole grains, and legumes.
* Keep your levels of vitamins B-1, B-6, B-12, C, and A, niacin, folic acid, calcium, magnesium, copper and iron sufficient. Use therapeutic doses to treat specific problems. Remember that high doses of B vitamins taken before bed can produce insomnia. Take these supplements before 6:00 PM. Amino acids work best if taken an hour or two before meals with fruit juice. Vitamin C with bioflavonoids and vitamin E can be taken at any time with other supplements. Remember that its usually not wise to take high amounts of just one vitamin or mineral. Balance is the key. Work out a program with a knowledgeable health care practitioner.

B vitamins: take 50 to 100 mg. at breakfast and at dinner. Use yeast free sources if you are allergic.
Folic acid: 400 mg. per day.
Magnesium: 500 mg. per day.
Vitamin C with bioflavonoids: 500 to 2000 mg. at breakfast and again at dinner.
Amino acids
    Tyrosine : 500 to 2500 mg. in the morning and mid-afternoon.
    Tryptophan: 500 to 4000 mg. at bedtime.
    Phenylalanine: 400 mg. per day.

Use pancreatic enzymes.
Take an acidophilus supplement every day to keep your intestinal flora healthy.
Take a good calcium/magnesium supplement. Make sure the calcium is a variety that is readily absorbable.
Use herbs judiciously for individual symptoms that accompany depression.

CELEBRATE:
It's Not All in Your Head!

*"Life is what we make it and the world is what we make
it. The eyes of the cheerful and of the melancholy man
are fixed upon the same creation; but very different are
the aspects which it bears to them."*

Albert Pike

Ann Landers once said, " One out of four people in this country is
mentally imbalanced. Think of your three closest friends...if they seem
okay, then, you're the one." If you're "the one" suffering from
depression, stop and rethink your dilemma. If we've learned anything
from our discussion it's that depression is a complex disease that is
directly impacted by nutritional, environmental and lifestyle factors.
That means that it can be cured by altering those same factors.

The full scope of the biochemistry of mood and behavior is just
beginning to emerge in scientific circles. The implications are
staggering. The simple truth is that everything we put in our mouths and
where and how we live determine our health and happiness to a great
degree. Look around, take an inventory of how you live and give your
body some support. Investigate your lifestyle and make some changes.

Questions raised from the information contained in this book are
worth investigating for yourself. In researching this book, one thing has
become extremely clear: innumerable factors including, what you eat,
how much light you live in, hormonal levels, the presence of infections,
exercise etc. all impact brain chemistry.

Inevitably, certain questions remain; Does a depressed mood initiate
changes in this biochemistry or is the opposite true. Perhaps the answer
lies in the elusive fact that the cause and effect of mood and chemistry
should be viewed as a continuous circle of biological reaction.
Everything we do, from gulping down a cup of coffee with a doughnut
to working in poorly lit environments can profoundly affect the delicate
biochemical balance of our bodies.

While we continue to explore the mysteries of the human body and
its psyche, remember that there already exists a substantial body of

evidence that natural medicine can effectively treat many forms of depression. That in itself is cause to celebrate.

THERE IS SO MUCH TO LEARN. EDUCATE YOURSELF.

It is in the area of naturopathy, which emphasizes the link between diet, environment and mental health that the best and safest potential cures for depression are found. The secret lies in finding out for yourself. Remember that even if your depression is the result of a sad event, nutritional and emotional support can only serve to help you better cope with your situation.

It is also vital to understand when approaching a complex disease like depression with natural medicine that there are individual differences in the way each person will respond to the treatments discussed in this book. What is essential is to locate a doctor or health care practitioner who is willing to work with natural therapies, and to tailor these therapies to fit your specific needs.

You might be asking yourself, if natural treatments for depression are as safe and effective as presented in this book, why don't more physicians recommend them. Generally speaking, the medical profession uses therapies that are familiar and considered standard treatments. Unfortunately, it takes a great deal of effort to test out alternative treatments and doctors usually don't take the time to investigate out of the ordinary therapies. As a result, if a doctor is not familiar with a particular treatment program such as using amino acids and vitamins to fight depression, he will probably be skeptical.

Natural medicine has never been taught in medical school. That fact does not, however, negate its value. The way we view disease and health will undergo dramatic changes during the 21st century. Doctors will have to educate themselves on the profound role that nutrition plays in the healing process. It's a sad fact that despite our economic status, the United States is an overmedicated, malnourished society which has forgotten the tried and true value of a healthy diet, herbs, vitamins and minerals.

Inevitably, the physician of the future will concentrate on the prevention of disease and its treatment through diet and natural supplementation. Thomas Edison foresaw this rebirth of natural medicine when he predicted, "The doctor of the future will give no medicine but will interest the patient in the care of the human frame, in diet and in the cause and prevention of disease."

The good news now is that depression is one of those diseases that can respond nicely to natural therapies. Like any healing therapy, treating depression with alternative medicine must be done with caution and supervision. Natural agents like vitamins, amino acids etc. may need to be added one at a time to assess their effectiveness. Dosages may have to be adjusted and patience is required to make objective evaluations of these treatment options.

Make a resolve now that you won't let your life be cheated or even worse, shortened by the "death wish" of depression. More importantly, don't be your own worst enemy. Jack Paar hit it on the head, "Looking back my life seems like one long obstacle race, with me as its chief obstacle."

If you want to get well naturally, arm yourself with the most effective natural tools and never give up. Remove the word impossible from your vocabulary and utilize the knowledge you have been given. Keep in mind that what may appear as today's miracle cure may be tomorrow's new scientific fact. Don't wait to find out. Don't blame yourself for feeling depressed. Look at depression the same way you would look at getting a fever or breaking out in hives and get yourself well. When you think about depression, always remember, it's not all in your head.

END NOTES

[1]Ann Blake Tracy. PROZAC PANACEA OR PANDORA, (Salt Lake City, Utah: Cassia Publications, 1994), 340.

[2]American Psychiatric Association. TEEN SUICIDE, (Washington D.C.: American Psychiatric Association, 1988), 4.

[3]Brian O'Reilly. "Depression and How To Beat It," FORTUNE, (November 29, 1993), 73.

[4]Ibid., 73.

[5]Patricia Slagle, M.D..THE WAY UP FROM DOWN, (New York: Random Books, 1987), 22.

[6]Simeon Margolis, M.D. and Peter V. Rabins, M.D.."Depression and Anxiety," THE JOHNS HOPKINS WHITE PAPERS, 1995, (Baltimore: The Johns Hopkins Institute, 1995), 16.

[7]Slagle, 10.

[8]Ibid., 70.

[9]Joe and Teresa Graedon. GRAEDON'S BEST MEDICINE FROM HERBAL REMEDIES TO HIGH TECH Rx BREAKTHROUGHS, (New York: Bantam Books, 1991), 213.

[10]Ibid., 211.

[11]Ibid., 212.

[12]Tracy, 83.

[13]Margolis, 16.

[14]Alan Gaby, M.D..THE DOCTOR'S GUIDE TO VITAMIN B-6, (Emmaus, Pennsylvania: Rodale Press, 1984), 62.

[15]Zoltan P. Rona, M.D..FIGHTING DEPRESSION, (St. Paul, Minnesota: Llewellyn Publications, 1994), 82.

[16]Linus Pauling. HOW TO LIVE LONGER AND FEEL BETTER, (New York: W.H. Freeman and Company, 1986), 195.

[17]Gaby, 63.

[18]PREVENTION'S NEW ENCYCLOPEDIA OF COMMON DISEASES. (Emmaus, Pennsylvania: Rodale Press, 1985), 232.

[19]Martin Zucker. "Food and Mood-There's No Mistaking the Connection," LET'S LIVE, (December, 1988), 12.

[20]Harvey Ross. FIGHTING DEPRESSION, (New Canaan,

Connecticut: Keats Publishing, 1992), 45.

[21]Tom Monte. WORLD MEDICINE THE EAST WEST GUIDE TO HEALING YOUR BODY, (New York: Putnam and Sons, 1993), 196.

[22]Richard J. and Judith J. Wurtman. "Carbohydrates and Depression," SCIENTIFIC AMERICAN, (January, 1989), 71.

[23]Monte, 197.

[24]Wurtman, 71.

[25]Ibid., 73.

[26]Slagle, 133.

[27]Ross, 51.

[28]Ibid., 28.

[29]Louise Tenney, "Herbs for Mental Illness," TODAY'S HERBS, (1986), 21.

[30]Ross, 30

[31]Robert C. Atkins, M.D..DR. ATKINS NUTRITION BREAKTHROUGH, (New York: William Morrow and Company, 1981), 97.

[32]Ibid., 98.

[33]Ross, 57.

[34]Oscar Janiger, M.D. and Philip Goldberg. A DIFFERENT KIND OF HEALING, (New York: Putnam and Sons, 1993), 71.

[35]PREVENTION'S NEW ENCYCLOPEDIA OF COMMON DISEASES, 232.

[36]Ibid., 231.

[37]Zucker, 14.

[38]Ross, 40

[39]PREVENTION'S NEW ENCYCLOPEDIA OF COMMON DISEASES, 223.

[40]Janiger, 72.

[41]PREVENTION'S NEW ENCYCLOPEDIA OF COMMON DISEASES, 230.

[42]Ibid., 228.

[43]Slagle, 70..

[44]Gaby, 63.

[45]Rona, 81.

[46]Slagle, 303.

[47]Michael T. Murray N.D.. NATURAL ALTERNATIVES TO OVER-THE-COUNTER AND PRESCRIPTION DRUGS, (New York; William Morrow and Company, 1994), 228.

[48]PREVENTION'S NEW ENCYCLOPEDIA OF COMMON DISEASES, 226.

[49]IBID., 226

[50]Mark S. Gold, M.D.. GOOD NEWS ABOUT DEPRESSION, (Toronto: Bantam Books, 1987), 123.

[51]Gaby, 64.

[52]Ibid., 66.

[53]PREVENTION'S NEW ENCYCLOPEDIA OF COMMON DISEASES, 229.

[54]Michael T. Murray, N.D. and Joseph E. Pizzorno, N.D..ENCYCLOPEDIA OF NATURAL MEDICINE, (Rocklin, California: Prima Publishing, 1991), 262.

[55]Gaby, 69.

[56]"Novel Pharmacologic Therapies in the Treatment of Experimental Traumatic Brain Injury, A Review," J. NEUROTRAUMA (United States: Fall, 1993), 215-61.

[57]PREVENTION'S NEW ENCYCLOPEDIA OF COMMON DISEASES, 228.

[58]Ibid., 229.

[59]Shari Lieberman M.A. and Nancy Bruning. DESIGN YOUR OWN VITAMIN AND MINERAL PROGRAM, (New York: Macmillan Publishing Company, 1988), 209.

[60]Atkins, 94.

[61]Gold, 123.

[62]PREVENTION'S NEW ENCYCLOPEDIA OF COMMON DISEASES, 239.

[63]Wurtman, 68.

[64]Angela Smyth. SEASONAL AFFECTIVE DISORDER, (London: Harper Collins Publishers, 1991), 85.

[65]Ibid., 40.

[66]Emrika Padus. THE COMPLETE GUIDE TO YOUR EMOTIONS AND YOUR HEALTH, (Emmaus, Pennsylvania: Rodale Press, 1992), 527.

[67]Wurtman, 68.

[68]Smyth, 83.

[69]PREVENTION'S NEW ENCYCLOPEDIA OF COMMON DISEASES, 234.

[70]Graedon, 206.

[71]Smyth, 213.

[72]Padus, 35.

[73]Janiger, 70.

[74]Norman Cousins. HEAD FIRST THE BIOLOGY OF HOPE, (New York: E.P. Dutton, 1987), 86.

[75]Ibid.

[76]Margolis, 6.

[77]Ibid.

[78]Colette Dowling. YOU MEAN I DON'T HAVE TO FEEL THIS WAY. (New York:Charles Scribner's Sons, 1991), 111.

[79]Ibid.

[80]Rona, 157.

[81]Elisa Lotter, Ph.D.. "Food and Mood," LET'S LIVE, (October, 1989), 54.

[82]Zucker, 17.

[83]Ibid., 18.

[84]Rona, 161.

[85]Atkins, 263.

[86]Zucker, 18.

[87]Gaby, 67.

[88]Zucker, 12.

[89]Alan Immerman. "Bad Bugs From a Bad Diet," VEGETARIAN TIMES, (January.February, 1980), 26.

[90]PREVENTION'S NEW ENCYCLOPEDIA OF COMMON DISEASES, 224.

[91]Rona, 135.

[92]PREVENTION'S NEW ENCYCLOPEDIA OF COMMON DISEASES, 238.

[93]William G. Crook, M.D. THE YEAST CONNECTION, (Jackson, Tennessee: Professional Books, 1986), 334.

[94]PREVENTION'S NEW ENCYCLOPEDIA OF COMMON DISEASES, 233.

[95]Margolis, 13.

[96]Andrew Weil, M.D.. NATURAL HEALTH, NATURAL MEDICINE. (Boston: Houghton Mifflin Company, 1990), 135.

[97]Annemarie Colbin. FOOD AND HEALING. (New York: Ballantine Books, 1986), 190.

[98]Marcia Starck. NATURAL HEALING, (St. Paul, Minnesota: Llewellyn Publications, 1993), 16. See, THE ART OF

AROMATHERAPY (New York: Destiny Books, 1977), 41.

[99]Tracy, 351.

[100]Murray, NATURAL ALTERNATIVES TO OVER-THE-COUNTER AND PRESCRIPTION DRUGS, 226.

[101]Ibid., 309.

[102]Ibid., 268.

[103]Ibid., 296.

BIBLIOGRAPHY

Adler, Jack. *"Biofeedback Physiological Means to Treat Depression,"* LET'S LIVE, January, 1982, 28-31.

Atkins, Robert C. M.D.. *DR. ATKINS NUTRITION BREAKTHROUGH.* New York: William Morrow and Company Inc., 1981.

Balch, James F., M.D. and Phyllis A. Balch C.N.C.. *PRESCRIPTION FOR NUTRITIONAL HEALING.* Garden City Park, New York: Avery Publishing Group, 1990.

Bricklin, Mark. *THE NATURAL HEALING ANNUAL* 1986. Emmaus, Pennsylvania: Rodale Press, 1986.

Bricklin, Mark. *THE NATURAL HEALING AND NUTRITION ANNUAL,* 1990. Emmaus, Pennsylvania: Rodale Press, 1990.

Chopra, Deepak M.D.. *QUANTUM HEALING EXPLORING THE FRONTIERS OF MIND/BODY MEDICINE.* New York: Bantam Books, 1989.

Colbin, Annemarie. *FOOD AND HEALING.* New York: Ballantine Books, 1986.

Cousins, Norman. *HEAD FIRST THE BIOLOGY OF HOPE.* New York: E.P. Dutton, 1987.

Crook, William G. M.D.. *THE YEAST CONNECTION, 3RD ED.* Jackson, Tennessee: Professional Books, 1986.

Dowling, Colette. *YOU MEAN I DON'T HAVE TO FEEL THIS WAY?.* NewYork: Charles Scribner's Sons, 1991.

Fitch, William Edward. *"Putrefactive Intestinal Toxemia,"* MEDICAL JOURNAL AND RECORDS, August 20, 1930, 183-187.

Gaby, Alan, M.D.. *THE DOCTOR'S GUIDE TO VITAMIN B-6.* Emmaus, Pennsylvania: Rodale Press, 1984.

Garrison, Robert H. Jr. M.A., R.Ph. and Elizabeth Somer, M.A.,R.D.. *THE NUTRITION DESK REFERENCE,* New Canaan, Connecticut: 1990.

Gold, Mark S. M.D.. *GOOD NEWS ABOUT DEPRESSION.* Toronto: Bantam Books, 1987.

Graedon, Joe and Teresa. *GRAEDONS BEST MEDICINE FROM HERBAL REMEDIES TO HIGH-TECH Rx BREAKTHROUGHS.* New York; Bantam Books, 1991.

Griffith, H. Winter M.D.. *COMPLETE GUIDE TO VITAMINS MINERALS & SUPPLEMENTS.* Tucson, Arizona: Fisher Books, 1988.

Hoffman, David. *SUCCESSFUL STRESS CONTROL THE NATURAL WAY.* Rochester, Vermont: Thorsons Publishers.

Immerman, Alan. *"Bad Bugs From a Bad Diet,"* VEGETARIAN TIMES, January/February 1980, 24-26.

Janiger, Oscar, M.D. and Philip Goldberg. *A DIFFERENT KIND OF HEALING.* New York: G.P. Putnam's Sons, 1993.

Lieberman, Shari, M.A., R.D. and Nancy Bruning. *DESIGN YOUR OWN VITAMIN AND MINERAL PROGRAM.* New York: Macmillan Publishing Company, 1988.

Lotter, Elisa Ph.D.. *"Food and Mood,"* LET'S LIVE, October, 1989,54-55.

Margolis, Simeon M.D., Ph.D. and Peter V. Rabins, M.D., M.P.H.. *"Depression and Anxiety,"* THE JOHNS HOPKINS WHITE PAPERS 1995, The Johns Hopkins Medical Institute, Baltimore, Maryland.

Monte, Tom. *WORLD MEDICINE THE EAST WEST GUIDE TO HEALING YOUR BODY.* New York: Putnam and Sons, 1993.

Morgan, Brain L.G. M.D.. *NUTRITION PRESCRIPTION.* New York: Crown Publishing, 1987.

Mowrey, Daniel B. Ph.D.. *HERBAL TONIC THERAPIES.* New Canaan, Connecticut: Keats Publishing, 1993.

Murray, Michael T. N.D., and Joseph E. Pizzorno, N.D.. *AN ENCYCLOPEDIA OF NATURAL MEDICINE.* Rocklin, California: Prima Publishing, 1991.

Murray, Michael T., N.D.. *NATURAL ALTERNATIVES TO OVER-THE-COUNTER AND PRESCRIPTION DRUGS.* New York: William Morrow and Company Inc., 1994.

Ody, Penelope. *THE COMPLETE MEDICINAL HERBAL.* New York: Dorling Kinderlsley, Inc., 1993.

O'Reilly, Brain. *"Depression and How to Beat It,"* FORTUNE, November 29, 1993, 70-78.

Padus, Emrika. *THE COMPLETE GUIDE TO YOUR EMOTIONS AND YOUR HEALTH.* Emmaus, Pennsylvania: Rodale Press, 1992.

Pauling, Linus. *HOW TO LIVE LONGER AND FEEL BETTER.* New York: W.H. Freeman and Company, 1986

PREVENTION'S NEW ENCYCLOPEDIA OF COMMON DISEASES.
Emmaus, Pennsylvania: Rodale Press, 1985.

Rona, Zoltan P. M.D.. *THE JOY OF HEALTH.* St. Paul, Minnesota:
Llewellyn Publications, 1994.

Ross, Harvey M. M.D.. *FIGHTING DEPRESSION.* New Canaan,
Connecticut: Keats Publishing, 1992.

Ryman, Danielle. *AROMATHERAPY.* New York: Bantam Books, 1993.

Satterlee, G. Reese M.D., and Watson W. Eldridge. *"Symptomatology of the Nervous System in Chronic Intestinal Toxemia,"* paper read at the Sixty-Eighth Annual Session of the American Medical Association, New York: June, 1917.

Scott, Julian and Susan. *NATURAL MEDICINE FOR WOMEN.* New York: Avon Books, 1991.

Siegel, Bernie S. M.D.. *LOVE MEDICINE & MIRACLES.* New York: Harper and Row, 1986.

Slagle, Patricia, M.D.. *THE WAY UP FROM DOWN.* New York: Random Books, 1987.

Smith, Janie Ph.D.. *"Sleep Deprivation Helps Treat Depression,"* LET'S LIVE, September, 1988, 79.

Smyth, Angela. *SEASONAL AFFECTIVE DISORDER.* Hammersmith, London: Harper Collins Publishers, 1991.

Starck, Marcia. *NATURAL HEALING.* St, Paul Minnesota: Llewellyn Publications, 1993.

Stein, Diane. *THE NATURAL REMEDY BOOK FOR WOMEN.* New York; The Crossing Press, 1992.

Tenney, Louise. *"Herbs for Mental Illness,"* TODAY'S HERBS, Woodland Books, 1986, 23-24.

Tenney, Louise M.H.. *MODERN DAY PLAGUES rev..* Pleasant Grove, Utah: Woodland Books, 1994.

Tenney, Louise. *"Nutrition and Mental Health,"* TODAY'S HERBS, Woodland Books, 1990, 27-28.

Tenney, Louise M.H.. *TODAY'S HERBAL HEALTH.* Pleasant Grove, Utah: Woodland Books, 1992.

Tracy, Ann Blake. *PROZAC PANACEA OR PANDORA.* Salt Lake City, Utah: Cassia Publications, 1994.

Wallis, Claudia. *"Why New Age Medicine is Catching On,"* TIME, November 4, 1991, vol. 138 No. 18, 68-76.

Weil, Andrew, M.D.. *NATURAL HEALTH, NATURAL MEDICINE.* Boston: Houghton Mifflin Company, 1990.

Wurtman, Richard J. and Judith J. *"Carbohydrates and Depression,"* SCIENTIFIC AMERICAN, January, 1989, 68-75.

Zucker, Martin. *"Food and Mood-There's No Mistaking The Connection,"* LET'S LIVE, December, 1988, 12-22.

INDEX